D0937374

the**facts**

Inflammatory bowel disease

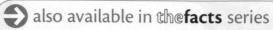

also available in the**facts** series

thefacts

Inflammatory bowel disease

LOUISE LANGMEAD
PETER IRVING

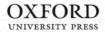

OXFORD
UNIVERSITY PRESS

OXFORD
UNIVERSITY PRESS

Great Clarendon Street, Oxford OX2 6DP

Oxford University Press is a department of the University of Oxford.
It furthers the University's objective of excellence in research, scholarship,
and education by publishing worldwide in

Oxford New York

Auckland Cape Town Dar es Salaam Hong Kong Karachi
Kuala Lumpur Madrid Melbourne Mexico City Nairobi
New Delhi Shanghai Taipei Toronto

With offices in

Argentina Austria Brazil Chile Czech Republic France Greece
Guatemala Hungary Italy Japan Poland Portugal Singapore
South Korea Switzerland Thailand Turkey Ukraine Vietnam

Oxford is a registered trade mark of Oxford University Press
in the UK and in certain other countries

Published in the United States
by Oxford University Press Inc., New York

© Oxford University Press, 2008

British Library Cataloguing in Publication Data

Data available

Library of Congress Cataloging in Publication Data

Langmead, Louise
  Inflammatory bowel disease: the facts/Louise Langmead, Peter Irving.
—The facts.
    p. cm.
  Includes index.
  ISBN 978–0–19–923071–6
1. Inflammatory bowel disease—Popular works. I. Irving, Peter, 1970– II. Title.
  RC862.I53L36 2008
  616.3'44—dc22

                                                                              2008023690

ISBN 978–0–19–923071–6

1 3 5 7 9 10 8 6 4 2

Typeset in Plantin
by Cepha Imaging Pvt. Ltd., Bangalore, India
Printed in Great Britain
by Ashford Colour Press Ltd., Gosport, Hampshire

Preface

Being asked to write a book aimed at providing information for people with IBD and their families was a great privilege. We have attempted to produce something that is readable and useful and which is complementary to the information that is available from other sources.

Although we have tried, wherever possible, to stick to the facts (as the title of the book demands) it is inevitable that in some areas we rely on conjecture and opinion. It is important to remember that opinion varies from person to person and doctor to doctor and, while we have done our best to be as balanced as possible, others are bound to disagree with some of our sentiments. Facts about IBD are largely realized through research. Research costs money and a proportion of that comes from patient support groups. The hard work and dedication of the members of organizations such as The National Association of Colitis and Crohn's Disease (NACC), The Crohn's and Colitis Foundation of America (CCFA), and the Australian Crohn's and Colitis Association (ACCA) is invaluable. Support of these groups by people with IBD, their families, and healthcare professionals is, therefore, vital. In buying this book you will be supporting the NACC as they are receiving the royalties.

PMI & LL, London, 2008

Acknowledgements

We would like to thank the following people for their contributions to this book. First and foremost, the people with IBD whose experiences are quoted in this book. Also, Della Hughes and Sue Catton who wrote the chapter on IBD nurse specialists. Finally, we would like to thank Deirdre Choo at the NACC for her helpful comments on the manuscript.

Contents

1

What is inflammatory bowel disease?

⮕ Key points

◆ Inflammatory bowel disease (IBD) is a group of conditions of which the commonest are ulcerative colitis and Crohn's disease.

◆ Others include IBD (unclassified), microscopic colitis, and pouchitis.

◆ There are several conditions that can cause similar symptoms to IBD but are not IBD. These include, infections, drug-induced colitis, coeliac disease, and irritable bowel syndrome.

Introduction

Inflammatory bowel disease (IBD) is exactly what it sounds like; a disease of the bowel that causes it to become inflamed. Specifically, IBD describes a chronic condition that may last for many years on and off, for which the cause is not yet fully understood.

Two main conditions are included under the heading of IBD. These are ulcerative colitis (UC) and Crohn's disease. There are also a number of other rarer conditions that may be classified as IBD (see Fig. 1.1).

There is much overlap between the different conditions both in the way they affect people, what they look like in the bowel, and their association with other conditions. There is also overlap among possible factors that probably contribute to the development of the different sorts of IBD, such as genes (see Chapter 2).

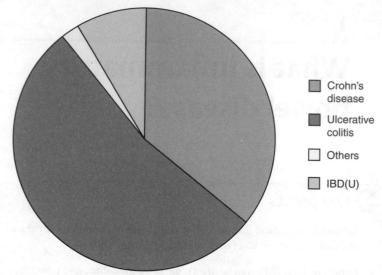

Crohn's disease

Ulcerative colitis

Others

IBD(U)

Figure 1.1 Conditions that make up inflammatory bowel disease.

The normal gut

In order to understand what happens when things go wrong in the gut it is worth spending some time learning about the healthy gut.

Terminology in the human gut can be confusing because there is often more than one word used for the same part. In order to understand how IBD affects the gut it is worth getting to know the anatomy of the human gut (what goes where and how it all joins up) and the function (what each bit is supposed to do). That way it is easier to appreciate how disease of different parts can cause quite different problems and symptoms.

Anatomy

The human gut is a long tube that starts at the mouth. Next comes the oesophagus, then the stomach, the small intestine, the large intestine, and, finally, the anus. The small intestine is made up of the duodenum, jejunum, and ileum. The large intestine is made up of the colon and rectum, which attaches to the anus. The gut is attached to various other organs along its course such as the liver and pancreas, which are important in allowing the gut to function normally.

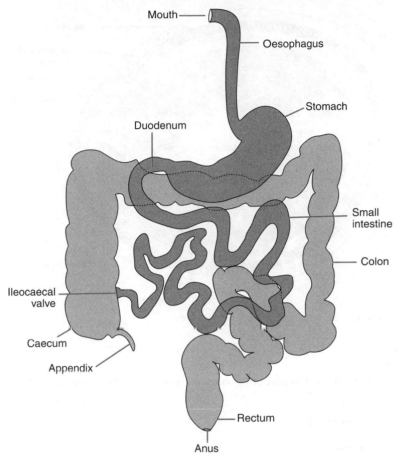

Figure 1.2 (a) The alimentary canal.

Function

The overall function of the gut is to get food into the body, to convert it into useful fuel to be delivered to the organs, and to dispose of the waste products. In other words, the gut functions rather like a power station; crude fuel is shovelled in at the top and is then refined into useful energy sources. The energy is fed down pipes to the bits that need it and the leftovers continue on to be jettisoned. However, the gut cannot do this alone. Other

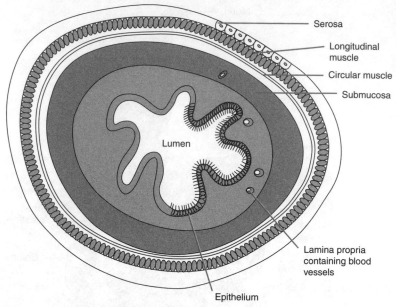

Figure 1.2 (b) The alimentary canal in cross-section.

organs are needed as part of the conversion of food to fuel (digestion). These are the:

◆ salivary glands

◆ pancreas

◆ liver

◆ gall bladder.

Once the food is processed and broken down, the products of digestion (sugars, amino acids, and fats) are absorbed through the gut lining into blood vessels surrounding the gut. They are then carried in the blood to other organs. What remains in the small intestine at the end of this process passes into the colon through the ileocaecal valve. At this point, the bowel content is liquid. However, as it passes along the colon, most of the water is reabsorbed through the bowel wall into the blood vessels. By the time the stool reaches the rectum it is, therefore, solid not liquid.

Malfunction

When any part of the gut becomes diseased this complicated process can go wrong in a variety of ways causing illness. This may result in symptoms in the affected organ, for example a stomach ulcer causing pain, or it may cause failure of energy production, for example, weight loss due to the malfunctioning of digestion. Symptoms of IBD will be discussed in more detail in Chapter 3.

Ulcerative colitis

UC is a condition in which part or all of the lining of the rectum and colon becomes inflamed and ulcerated. Although inflammation and ulceration of the bowel can occur for a variety of reasons, such as dysentery or as a side effect of radiotherapy, by definition, the cause in UC is not known (see Chapter 2).

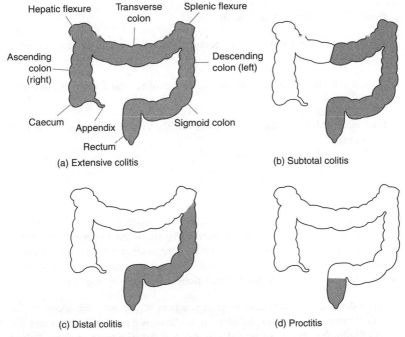

Figure 1.3 The extent of colitis.

What happens to ulcerative colitis over time?

The disease can affect anyone at any time. It is a chronic condition, that is to say long lasting. The inflammation may wax and wane either with or without treatment so that a typical pattern of flare up or relapse occurs between periods of calm or remission.

How much of the bowel is affected in ulcerative colitis

The pattern of UC in the bowel is very typical. It (nearly) always affects the rectum and then extends up the colon to a differing degree in each individual. For most patients what you start with is what you end up with. In other words if you have left-sided colitis at diagnosis it is not very likely to become more extensive as time goes on or with subsequent flare ups. However, in some people, the disease can become more extensive over time. It is still unclear how often this happens. It is thought that about 1 in 10 patients with proctitis develop subtotal colitis within 10 years of diagnosis.

Disease extent in ulcerative colitis

Proctitis = rectum only inflamed

Distal colitis = left-sided colitis: rectum, sigmoid and descending colon inflamed

Subtotal colitis = rectum, sigmoid, descending and transverse colon inflamed

Extensive colitis = pan colitis, total colitis: entire colon and rectum inflamed

---

Crohn's disease

Crohn's disease is less easy to classify than UC because it is more variable in what it affects and how. It was first described by and named after Burrill Crohn, an American gastroenterologist, in 1932. The disease is now recognized to cover a wide variety of presentations and patterns of gut inflammation. The typical features of Crohn's disease may occur separately or together.

Crohn's disease can cause problems in any part of the gut from ulcers in the mouth to abscesses around the anus. It is classically patchy so that there are areas of inflammation interspersed with normal gut. However, in about half of people with Crohn's disease, the area affected is limited to the last bit of the small bowel and some, or all of the large bowel. When Crohn's disease affects the large bowel only (Crohn's colitis), it can sometimes be difficult to distinguish it from UC (see below).

Crohn's disease may affect only the internal lining (mucosa) of the gut (like UC) or the inflammation can go deeper into the bowel wall causing a perforation or fistula to form. This can allow bowel contents to leak outside the gut causing collections of infection (abscesses) to develop.

A fistula is an abnormal channel causing a connection between two surfaces that are not normally linked, e.g. between the gut lumen and the skin. These occur in approximately one-third of patients with Crohn's disease at

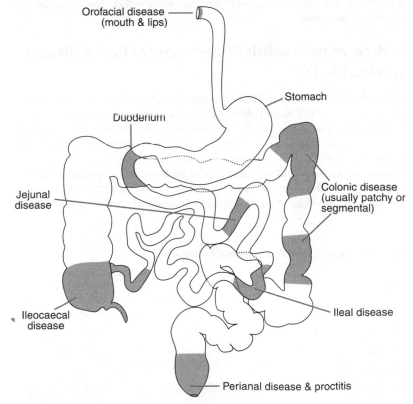

Figure 1.4 Common sites affected by Crohn's disease. One or more site may be affected in any individual.

some point in their lives. The commonest place to develop fistulas is around the anus.

Another complication of Crohn's disease occurs when the bowel lumen becomes narrowed causing blockages. These narrowings are called strictures. They develop as a result of healing and scarring in the bowel wall after inflammation resolves.

See Figure 3.1 in Chapter 3.

Some people are more prone to inflammatory type Crohn's causing ulceration and bleeding of the gut mucosa, whereas some are more prone to 'penetrating' disease that causes abscesses, perforations, and fistula formation. Others seem to be more likely to have stricturing disease. Some people have more than one type of Crohn's disease at the same time and some will change from one type to another over time.

Indeterminate colitis/inflammatory bowel disease unclassified

When the inflammation in IBD is confined to the colon it could be due to either UC or Crohn's disease. Although these conditions are distinct in several ways, as described in this and the next chapter, there are times when it can be very difficult to make a firm diagnosis of either. This can be especially true when the condition is newly diagnosed and in its early stages. Sometimes, despite several tests and repeated sets of biopsies, your specialist may tell you that they are not sure whether you have UC or Crohn's colitis. This is known as IBD (unclassified), although it is sometimes called indeterminate

Table 1.1 Types of Crohn's disease and frequency

Site	Patients (%)
Ileocolonic	45
Colonic only	25
Terminal ileum only	20
Extensive small bowel	5
Perianal only	3
Other (oral, gastroduodenal only)	2

colitis. Usually, over the next year or two, the diagnosis becomes clearer. For example, the disease pattern might change to be more like Crohn's by affecting another part of the gut or the perianal region. Alternatively, a complication seen more commonly in UC may appear (e.g. primary sclerosing cholangitis see Chapter 12).

Although not knowing the exact diagnosis can be frustrating, as long as the disease is under control, there are no drawbacks to it being unclassified.

However, if the disease cannot be controlled with drugs and surgery is required, a problem can arise. This is because the long-term surgical options depend on whether the underlying diagnosis is UC or Crohn's disease. If the diagnosis is unclear and you require surgery, your surgeon and gastroenterologist will recommend you have a subtotal colectomy (see Chapter 9). This leaves you with the future option of either a pouch or an ileorectal anastomosis. After surgery the colon is examined carefully by the pathologist. With such a large specimen it is often possible to make a firm diagnosis. However, occasionally even after the whole colon has been examined under the microscope, it is still not possible to make a diagnosis one way or the other. In this case the disease is labelled indeterminate colitis. Experience tells us that people with this condition tend to have a higher incidence of pouchitis and problems after reconstructive surgery than people with UC. This is because a proportion actually have Crohn's disease, which normally recurs in pouches (see Chapter 9).

Others

Microscopic colitis: collagenous colitis, lymphocytic colitis

Microscopic colitis is a condition that causes watery diarrhoea without bleeding. There are two main sorts of microscopic colitis; collagenous colitis and lymphocytic colitis. The cause is not known but some drugs (e.g. diclofenac) have been implicated. The lining of the bowel looks normal during colonoscopy but biopsy samples show a typical pattern of inflammation under the microscope. In collagenous colitis, this consists of an increase in the thickness of the layer of collagen found in the bowel wall. In lymphocytic colitis, increased numbers of lymphocytes are found in the bowel wall.

Unlike UC and Crohn's disease, microscopic colitis tends to occur in late middle age and is more common in women. Sometimes the condition gets better spontaneously, although treatment may be required. It is a rarer condition than IBD.

Diversion colitis

Diversion colitis is inflammation in a section of the bowel that no longer has faeces flowing through it, i.e. the faeces have been diverted. For example, if the colon has been removed with formation of an ileostomy, the rectum is often left in place but is simply closed off at its upper end (see Chapter 9). Therefore, no faeces flow through the rectum. Commonly the lining of the rectum becomes mildly inflamed. Sometimes, however, it can be severely inflamed causing passage of blood and mucus through the anus. This kind of colitis disappears if the bowel is rejoined and the stream of faeces restored.

Diversion colitis can occur in any individual having surgery for any condition (i.e. it is not specific for people with IBD and may occur if you have colonic surgery for cancer or another reason). This suggests that something in the faeces is needed to keep the bowel healthy and that diversion colitis is not part of the IBD spectrum.

Pouchitis

Pouchitis is inflammation that occurs in the pouch after pouch surgery (see Chapter 9). This condition usually occurs in people who have had a colectomy for IBD but not those who have had it for polyps or other reasons. This suggests that it is part of the spectrum of IBD.

What is not inflammatory bowel disease?

Infection

Infections with bacteria, viruses, or parasites can lead to inflammation of the gut that may look very similar to IBD. The distinction is that in the case of infection, the gut returns to normal once the bug has been eradicated by the immune system or by treatment. The condition does not recur unless another infection is caught. For example, *Campylobacter* is a bacterium that can cause a colitis in healthy people. If treated appropriately they recover completely with no lasting damage to the gut. Of course, people with IBD can catch infections too and, in fact, up to 1 in 5 of flare ups of UC may be provoked by infections.

Drug-induced gut inflammation

Some medications can cause inflammation in the gut that can look similar to IBD, e.g. non-steroidal anti-inflammatory drugs (e.g. ibuprofen, naproxen) and some potassium supplement tablets can cause ulceration and bleeding in the gut. Once the drug is stopped, the inflammation improves, which helps to distinguish drug-induced inflammation from IBD. Non-steroidal anti-inflammatory drugs, like Crohn's disease, can cause strictures in the gut.

Of course, many drugs, such as antibiotics, can cause disturbance in gut function leading to symptoms, such as bloating and diarrhoea but only rarely do they cause actual inflammation.

Coeliac disease

This condition is caused by a specific immune reaction to gluten, which is a protein found in wheat. When affected patients eat wheat the immune system reacts against it and causes inflammation in the small intestine. This leads to malabsorption of nutrients. The inflammation can be cured by avoiding gluten in the diet.

Irritable bowel syndrome and functional gut disorders

These conditions are characterized by a variety of gut-related symptoms such as diarrhoea, bloating, constipation, and abdominal pain. Other symptoms, such as tiredness, are also commonly found in people with irritable bowel syndrome (IBS) or functional gut disorders. However, unlike in IBD, in IBS there is no obvious bowel inflammation or pathological abnormality of the gut. IBS is very common, affecting up to 1 in 5 people during their lifetime. Normally, the condition is mild and self-limiting, but it can cause severe symptoms in some people.

IBS and functional gut disorders do not cause ulceration or bleeding or affect absorption of nutrients across the gut wall. Therefore they do not usually cause weight loss or anaemia.

Many patients with UC or Crohn's disease will also suffer with IBS at some time or other (see Chapter 4). Indeed, the crossover of symptoms makes it difficult to distinguish between the two (IBD and IBS) at times.

Conclusions

IBD is a spectrum of conditions of unknown cause that result in inflammation in the bowel. The commonest forms of IBD are Crohn's disease and UC.

2

Who gets inflammatory bowel disease and why?

> **➔ Key points**
>
> ◆ The three main components that contribute to the development of inflammatory bowel disease (IBD) are our genes, our environment, and our inflammatory response.
>
> ◆ IBD is relatively common affecting about 1 in every 250 people.
>
> ◆ The incidence of IBD is increasing.

Introduction: Why do people develop inflammatory bowel disease?

One of the commonest questions we get asked by people who have recently been diagnosed with inflammatory bowel disease (IBD) is 'Why did I get it?'. However, IBD does not have a single cause. We know that there are three important components to the development of IBD. First, people who develop IBD have to have inherited the right genes. However, having these genes is not enough by itself to cause IBD. To develop the condition, people with IBD also need to encounter a trigger, or perhaps several triggers, called environmental factors (see box on p 15). Exactly what these triggers are is poorly understood and they may vary from person to person. Finally, we also know that the bacteria in our intestines play a part in causing inflammation in the bowel wall and the development of IBD.

How common is IBD?

The diagnosis of ulcerative colitis (UC) and, in particular of Crohn's disease has increased markedly over the last 50 years. Today, in the UK, Crohn's

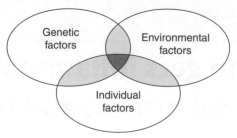

Figure 2.1 Why do people develop IBD?

affects about 1–2 per 1000 people and UC about 2–3 per 1000. Every year about 1 in 10 000 people is newly diagnosed with UC and a similar number with Crohn's. Although these numbers may sound small, this amounts to about 200 000 people with IBD in the UK and about 12 000 new cases every year.

Age and gender distribution

IBD can present at any age but is most commonly diagnosed in young adulthood, between the ages of 15 and 40. There tends to be a second peak later in life between the ages of about 60 and 80. In general, both conditions are as common in men as they are in women.

Is inflammatory bowel disease found in all countries?

There is a marked variation around the world in the occurrence of IBD. Both UC and Crohn's are more common in industrialized nations than in developing countries. However, things seem to be changing. Both UC and Crohn's are becoming more common in developing countries, for reasons that are not entirely clear.

Although our genes clearly play a part (see below) other factors are probably involved. For example, migration from countries where IBD is uncommon to areas where it is more common leads to an increased chance of getting IBD. This suggests that an 'environmental' factor in the new country is involved in the development of IBD.

What is meant by an 'environmental' factor?

An environmental factor is any non-genetic factor. Examples include smoking, diet, exposure to infections, exercise habits, or even something as simple as the climate in which we live.

What causes inflammatory bowel disease?

Despite years of intensive research the cause of IBD is not fully understood. Of course, particularly with the advent of the World Wide Web, it is possible to find people who will tell you that *they* have discovered the cause. Some will even offer to cure your IBD, normally in exchange for a considerable amount of money! However, in reality things are not that simple. Nevertheless, major advances in the understanding of the causes of IBD have been made over the last few years and our knowledge about the causes of IBD increases year by year.

Genetic factors (genes)

Humans have about 30 000 genes. These genes, combined with other factors, are responsible for determining what we look like and what illnesses we get. We all have two copies of every gene, one from each of our parents.

The importance of genes in IBD first became apparent when studies showed that relatives of people with IBD were more likely to develop the condition themselves. Extensive research over the last few years has helped to unravel the genetics of IBD. This is potentially a very exciting area of research and it is hoped that it will lead to advances both in our understanding of how and why IBD occurs, and also in its treatment. However, this is not a simple process. Neither Crohn's disease nor UC are 'single gene disorders' like cystic fibrosis, which is caused by a problem in a single gene. Both Crohn's and UC have been linked with many genes, with more being found regularly. *IBD1* was the first such gene to be discovered and is linked to Crohn's disease.

The contribution of these genes to the development of IBD is, however, relatively small. For example, someone with two copies of the high-risk version of the *IBD1* gene (one from each parent) is between 20 and 40 times more likely to develop Crohn's disease than somebody with two low-risk copies. However, they still only have about a 1 in 30 chance of developing Crohn's. Put another way, over 95% of people with two copies of the high-risk version do not develop Crohn's disease.

In this way, Crohn's disease and UC are similar to many other conditions, such as diabetes and schizophrenia, which have a genetic component, probably from several different genes, but also require interaction with the environment.

If I have inflammatory bowel disease, will my children get it?

Again, this is a common concern of people with IBD, and understandably so. We know that IBD runs in families but that genes are only part of the problem. Therefore, giving accurate estimates of the risk of a relative of someone with IBD developing the condition is difficult. Crohn's disease runs in families more than UC, and the chance of developing IBD is higher for closer relatives than distant ones. Certain racial groups, such as Jews, have a higher incidence of IBD.

Of first degree relatives, siblings (brothers and sisters) are at the highest risk of also getting IBD. Next come parents of someone with IBD, and last children. A sibling or child of someone with Crohn's disease is said to be 20–40 times more likely to develop IBD than a member of the general population. However, this only equates to an overall risk of about 1 in 15. Therefore, 90–95% of brothers or sisters of someone with IBD will not get it. For UC, the risk is less. In the situation where both parents have IBD, their children have about a 1 in 3 chance of also developing IBD. It is important to understand that these figures are *very* rough estimates.

A good illustration of the fact that genes are important in IBD comes from studying identical twins. Identical twins are exact genetic copies of each other. If one twin develops Crohn's disease, the other has about a 50% chance of getting it too. Of course, if the development of IBD was entirely due to genes, you would expect that if one twin has IBD then the other would always get it too. However, the fact that they don't tells us something—other factors must be involved.

Environmental factors

A problem with many studies showing associations between IBD and environmental factors is that they cannot show whether a factor *causes* the disease or whether it is simply linked to it. For example, if we were to perform a study to see if riding a bicycle protected against developing lung cancer, we may find a positive association because people who ride bikes are less likely to smoke, not because cycling prevents lung cancer. Although statistical tests can help get around this, confounding factors, as they are called, are an inherent problem with this kind of research.

Smoking

Surprisingly, there is a strong link between smoking and IBD. Although the effects are well described, they are incompletely understood. UC is generally a disease of non-smokers. Only 1 in 8 people with UC smoke compared with about 1 in 4 of the general population in the UK. There is also a link between giving up smoking and developing UC for the first time or suffering a relapse. However, the general health risks of smoking, such as cancer and heart disease, are so serious that the fear of UC should not discourage people from giving up smoking.

In contrast, Crohn's is a disease of smokers, with some studies showing that more than half of people with Crohn's disease smoke. Smoking doubles the risk of getting Crohn's disease. The effects seem to be more pronounced in women than in men. The reason why Crohn's is associated with smoking, and UC with non-smoking, is not clear, although many theories have been suggested. These include that smoking: (1) alters the quality of mucus produced by the bowel (mucus protects the lining of the bowel); (2) alters the way the bowel contracts; (3) alters blood supply to the gut; (4) has effects on the immune system; and (5) has a direct effect on inflammation within the bowel itself.

Effects of smoking in Crohn's disease

◆ Increases the risk of developing Crohn's disease

◆ Makes it more active

◆ Makes medications used to treat Crohn's less effective

◆ Makes recurrence of the disease after surgery worse

Whatever the mechanism, we know that smoking makes Crohn's disease worse. For example compared with non-smokers, smokers with Crohn's disease have worse symptoms and are more likely to need treatment with drugs such as azathioprine. Smoking also doubles the likelihood of needing further operations after having had surgery for Crohn's disease and, finally, smoking also decreases the effectiveness of some treatments.

Most importantly, stopping smoking is an effective treatment for active Crohn's and decreases the chance of having a disease flare by more than 50%.

Put another way, stopping smoking is about as effective as starting azathioprine. It probably also decreases the chance of *ever* needing surgery. The beneficial effects of giving up smoking occur fairly rapidly and are long lasting, with ex-smokers having similar risks of relapse as those who have never smoked.

Overall, therefore, all people with Crohn's who smoke should stop. It's never too late! (See also Chapter 14.)

Dietary causes

The role dietary factors play in causing IBD is less clear than for smoking and genetics. In view of the fact that IBD affects the gut, it is not surprising that both people with IBD and those who study the disease have wondered whether something we eat may play a part in causing IBD. There are many possible culprits.

Several studies have suggested that **breast feeding** may protect against developing IBD. The length of time for which breast feeding occurs may also be important (benefits up to 1 year have been suggested). Some people have suggested that this effect may be related to delaying exposure to **cow's milk**.

Intake of **sugar and refined carbohydrate** (processed foods such as white bread and white rice) has been linked with both UC and Crohn's. However, it is possible that a higher intake of sugar and refined carbohydrate may be a result of IBD rather than a cause. Alternatively, diets high in these substances are found chiefly in the developed world, and may simply be confounding factors.

The role of dietary **fibre** is not clear. Some studies have shown that fibre intake is lower in patients with IBD. However, this might be because it could worsen symptoms in people with active disease (see Chapter 12).

The role of **fat**, particularly chemically processed hydrogenated fats such as margarine, has also been investigated. This was in part prompted by the geographical distribution of Crohn's and UC, and the fact that IBD was first recognized around the time that margarine was introduced into Western diets. Further studies examining an association between IBD and margarine have produced conflicting results as have those examining the relative contributions of **saturated** and **unsaturated fats**. Similarly, **fast food**, which is typically high in fat, has been linked with IBD, again without any definite evidence emerging.

In summary, no definite dietary cause for IBD has been found and most doctors who specialize in IBD do not believe that it is caused by something that we eat. It is, however, possible that there may be something in the diet that, at least for some people, triggers IBD. The role of diet, however, can be important in managing the symptoms of IBD and is discussed in Chapter 12.

Medications

A link between Crohn's and the **oral contraceptive pill (OCP)** has been debated for some time. Studies have shown that women who take the OCP are about twice as likely to have Crohn's as those who do not. However, whether the OCP is a causative or confounding factor is unknown. It may be reasonable to try an alternative form of contraception if you think that your Crohn's is being made worse by the OCP.

Non-steroidal anti-inflammatory drugs (NSAIDs) are commonly used as pain killers. Many of these drugs, such as diclofenac, require a prescription, but others, such as ibuprofen, are available for purchase at pharmacies. Although some patients with IBD are able to tolerate these medications, others find that they cause their disease to flare or that they worsen their symptoms. In general, patients with IBD should probably avoid NSAIDs if possible. However, if they are used they should be used sparingly.

Infections

An infective cause of either Crohn's or UC has been sought for some time. Although most researchers have felt that a single infective cause for either disease is unlikely, it is important to keep an open mind. Of all the potentially infective organisms that have been suggested as causes of IBD two stand out, not least because they have both been associated with a certain amount of controversy.

In the 1990s when the **measles virus** and the **measles, mumps and rubella (MMR) vaccine** were first proposed as possible causes of Crohn's disease, a 'lively debate' resulted. Understandably, some parents became concerned about having their children vaccinated. Unfortunately, this created a real possibility of outbreaks of these potentially serious infections.

This theory was based on two studies. The first apparently showed that measles virus was present in the bowel of some people with Crohn's disease. The second described 12 children with a form of autism associated with IBD. The parents of all these children felt that their symptoms were related to receiving the MMR vaccine and a possible link was therefore suggested. Many readers will be familiar with the consequences of the publication of these papers and of the different interpretations made of them. Perhaps because the research originated in the UK, the impact was much greater there than in most other countries that use MMR.

Fortunately, the situation is now much clearer. The majority of subsequent studies have failed to find measles virus in Crohn's patients. Several large publications have examined the role of MMR in Crohn's disease and none has identified a link.

Mycobacterium avium paratuberculosis, also known as **MAP**, is known to cause a disease in cattle called Johne's disease. Johne's disease is very similar to Crohn's disease and some people believe that Crohn's in humans is caused by MAP. Cattle with Johne's disease produce milk containing MAP and, although cows with obvious disease are removed from the milk herd, some animals can be infected without displaying symptoms. Pasteurization does not eliminate MAP entirely and there is little doubt that those of us who drink milk are exposed to MAP.

The theory that MAP causes Crohn's disease is supported by the fact that some studies have found MAP in either blood samples or pieces of inflamed intestine taken from people with Crohn's. However, MAP has also been found in samples from people with UC and also from people without any bowel disease (healthy controls). When the results of all studies are pooled together, MAP is found in similar numbers of people whether they have Crohn's, UC, or are healthy controls.

Overall, therefore, there is no conclusive evidence that MAP causes Crohn's disease. It is, however, possible that in a small subset of people MAP may make Crohn's disease worse or even be the cause of their disease. Equally, MAP may turn out to be yet another red herring. Research continues into the role of MAP in IBD and we hope that this will help clear up some or all of these unanswered questions. For information regarding anti-MAP therapy as a treatment for Crohn's disease see Chapter 11.

The appendix

People who have had their appendix removed, particularly if it was done before the age of 20, seem to be protected against developing UC. It has also been suggested that people who have had their appendix removed who do develop UC have a milder form of the disease than those who still have their appendix. Although the reason for this association is unclear, it seems that the appendix is involved in the immune response. Occasionally people have even undergone surgery to remove their appendix as a treatment for UC; the results of this are discussed in Chapter 11.

Hygiene theory

The fact that IBD is more common in the West prompted the theory that an increase in standards of hygiene might somehow predispose people to IBD.

The thinking behind this relates to the development of the immune system. As sanitation standards increase, children are exposed to fewer infections and encounter them later in life. However, why infections should protect against IBD is unclear, but similar associations have been seen with asthma and multiple sclerosis.

Stress and inflammatory bowel disease

Some people find that stress can exacerbate the symptoms of IBD. Of course, many people, whether they have IBD or not, find that their bowel habit changes when they are under stress. This is a normal response and is best demonstrated by the number of people who need to rush to the toilet before exams or interviews.

However, some people with IBD find that stress actually causes their disease to flare up. Recent work in this area has shown that stress can worsen inflammation in the bowels. Of course, this does not mean that IBD is caused solely by stress but simply that in some people stress may play a part in exacerbating IBD. Of course, removing all stress from life is impossible, but perhaps relaxation techniques and/or hypnotherapy (see Chapter 7) may prove to be helpful for such people.

Deficiency in inflammatory response

The third important aspect of the development of IBD relates to the way our immune system works and there is a theory that Crohn's disease is caused by a deficiency in the inflammatory response.

When bacteria escape from the lumen of the bowel into the bowel wall, the immune system rapidly kills the bacteria. However, in Crohn's disease this response may be ineffective allowing the bacteria to survive causing a prolonged inflammatory response. This fascinating theory, if proved correct might revolutionize the way we treat Crohn's disease. However, the jump from proposing theories to developing effective treatments is enormous and generally takes years if not decades.

The role of bacteria in our guts

There are more bacteria in our gastrointestinal tract than there are cells in our body. The 100 000 000 000 000 (or so!) bacteria that live in our bowels are made up of several hundred different species. They are mostly in the colon and perform a variety of important roles in our bodies including aiding digestion and helping to prevent infections by pathogenic (disease-causing) bacteria. However, we are now starting to understand that these bacteria are also important in the development of IBD. In particular, the way which they interact with the immune system in the gut seems to play a vital role in causing inflammation.

Probiotics, sometimes also known as 'friendly bacteria', are being studied as a treatment for IBD and are helping us to understand how altering the balance of the different bacterial species in the gut can improve inflammation (see Chapter 12).

Conclusions

We hope that this chapter has helped to explain the factors that may be involved in the development of IBD. It seems likely that different factors are involved for different people, which, considering that IBD represents a range of diseases, is not surprising. Nevertheless, while research continues in these areas, our understanding of these conditions and the potential for new treatments increases.

3

Gut symptoms of inflammatory bowel disease

➔ Key points

- ◆ Inflammatory bowel disease causes a variety of gut symptoms.

- ◆ Ulcerative colitis causes bloody diarrhoea with mucus and abdominal pain due to inflammation in the colon.

- ◆ Crohn's disease may cause diarrhoea, weight loss, abdominal pain, and vomiting due to intestinal or colonic inflammation.

- ◆ Strictures, perianal disease, and fistulas can complicate Crohn's disease.

Introduction

All patients with inflammatory bowel disease (IBD) get gastrointestinal symptoms when their disease is active. However, these symptoms vary depending on which part of the gut is affected, how it is affected, and how active the disease is.

People with IBD may also experience a variety of other symptoms. These include general symptoms, such as tiredness and lethargy, and symptoms caused by inflammation in organs other than the gut, so-called extraintestinal (outside the gut) manifestations. General symptoms are discussed in Chapter 4 and extraintestinal symptoms in Chapter 13.

Ulcerative colitis

Common symptoms of ulcerative colitis

- *Diarrhoea*: loose stools

- *Bowel frequency*: the need to open your bowels more often than usual

- *Urgency*: the need to get to the toilet quickly

- *Blood*: with active disease, blood may appear in the stools

- *Mucus*: when the bowel is inflamed, mucus, a jelly-like substance, can sometimes be seen in the stool

- *Abdominal pain*: cramping pain often associated with going to the toilet.

When ulcerative colitis (UC) is active, the lining of the bowel becomes inflamed and ulcerated. This stops it from functioning normally. As one of the main jobs of the colon is to reabsorb water, when it stops working properly the stool is more fluid, resulting in diarrhoea.

The urge to go to the toilet is induced by faeces moving from the colon into the rectum. The muscles of the anus help to keep the stool in the rectum until we are able to reach a toilet. However, when people have diarrhoea, liquid stool moves into the rectum more frequently than normal formed stool would. As it is liquid, it is harder to hold on to. Therefore, not only do people with active IBD need to go to the toilet more frequently than usual, they may also need to get there very quickly, a symptom known as urgency. If this is very severe, people may occasionally have episodes of incontinence (accidents).

People with active IBD may also have trouble distinguishing whether they need to pass wind or stool. This is because the rectum, although very good at telling the difference between solid and gas (which allows people to pass wind without fear of soiling themselves) is not good at distinguishing between liquid and gas. This can result in very frequent trips to the toilet for people with diarrhoea.

With active inflammation, the bowel wall may increase its production of mucus and may also leak blood and pus. Therefore, as well as being loose, the bowel motions may contain blood, mucus, and pus. With active inflammation of the colon, cramping pains in the tummy can be very severe and are probably caused by contractions of the inflamed bowel. They are often worst immediately before or after defecation (see below for pain caused by strictures).

Some people notice that their wind and stools are particularly odorous when their IBD is active. This is a common symptom that usually improves as the inflammation gets better.

How does disease activity and extent affect symptoms?

The sort of symptoms you get differ according to how much of the bowel is affected (the extent of colitis) (Chapter 1, Fig. 1.3). The extent of inflammation and its severity will also affect how you feel. However, the extent of colitis does not necessarily tally with how severe the disease is. For example, you could have severe proctitis or mild pancolitis. When the inflammation is severe it tends to cause worse symptoms, with very frequent motions. Often this will continue through the night so that you are woken from sleep by the need to go to the toilet. There may also be a lot of blood, sometimes without any stool. You could also become feverish and have persistent abdominal pain.

Proctitis

As proctitis only affects the rectum, the rest of the colon (i.e. 80–90%) is unaffected and still functions normally. Therefore, people with active proctitis may not get diarrhoea at all. In fact they may suffer from constipation. In this situation, treating the constipation can sometimes improve the proctitis. People with proctitis normally get bleeding that is bright red and may be mixed with mucus.

When the inflammation in the rectum is severe, it can become very irritated. This can result in the need to go to the toilet frequently to pass a mixture of blood and mucus with little or no stool.

Table 3.1 Typical symptoms of active ulcerative colitis determined by disease location

Proctitis	Urgency, bright red blood and mucus. Some solid stools. Sometimes constipation
Left-sided colitis, distal colitis	Bloody diarrhoea, left-sided abdominal pain, dark blood mixed with stool
Subtotal colitis/pancolitis	Frequent watery diarrhoea with blood and mucus. Abdominal pain, fever and weight loss

Left-sided colitis, distal colitis

With disease affecting more of the colon but limited to the left side, diarrhoea becomes more predominant. Severe attacks cause bloody diarrhoea. The blood is often darker than in people with proctitis as it comes from higher up in the bowel. People with distal colitis may also get cramping pain in the tummy especially on the left side.

Subtotal and pancolitis

Disease that affects most of the colon invariably causes diarrhoea. When the inflammation is severe, people may have diarrhoea as often as 20 times per day. Other signs of a severe attack include fevers, abdominal pain, and weight loss. As with distal colitis, milder attacks may cause diarrhoea or looser stool without blood.

As mentioned in Chapter 1, UC is a relapsing remitting disease. This means there are periods of time when it is inactive with few symptoms and people feel fairly or completely normal. These are interspersed with periods of active disease when symptoms come back. Spontaneous improvement of symptoms can occur without treatment. Obviously the aim of treatment is to minimize the symptoms during the active phase and speed up the return to the inactive phase. Treatment is also used to maintain remission and reduce the frequency of relapses once the inflammation has resolved. Although remission can occur spontaneously, it is important to note that severe attacks are very unlikely to resolve without any treatment.

Recognizing a relapse of ulcerative colitis

All people experience some irregularities in their bowel habit (frequency, consistency of stools, urgency) from time to time so it can be difficult to tell whether a change is the beginning of a relapse of UC or is just a normal variation. However, most people with UC are very good at recognizing when a relapse is starting. The key things to look out for are:

◆ increased frequency

◆ getting up at night

◆ bleeding

◆ associated extraintestinal manifestations (see Chapter 13).

These symptoms are suggestive of increasing activity of inflammation. If they do not settle down after a couple of days you should consult a doctor.

Living with inflammatory bowel disease

Urgency and wind are embarrassing problems. Trying to act naturally while holding on until you can find a toilet is a horrible situation for anyone. People with IBD have to live with this situation all too frequently. Many also say that their wind and diarrhoea have a very bad smell. This makes them embarrassed to use communal toilets and sometimes even to venture out of their house.

Although there is no obvious remedy to this, if you cast your mind back to the last time you went to the outpatient clinic, it might help to think that many patients there suffer the same anxiety.

Crohn's disease

Common symptoms of Crohn's disease

◆ *Pain*: abdominal pain in Crohn's can occur for a number of reasons. It is often crampy.

◆ *Diarrhoea*: there are several reasons why people with Crohn's disease get diarrhoea. If Crohn's affects the colon the diarrhoea may be bloody.

◆ *Weight loss*: poor appetite and malabsorption of nutrients can cause weight loss.

◆ *Fever*: this can result from abscesses or bowel inflammation.

◆ *Perianal abscesses/discharge*: fistulas and abscesses around the anus affect about 1 in 3 people with Crohn's disease.

◆ *Poor growth/delayed puberty*: poor nutrition and active inflammation can both contribute to poor growth and delayed puberty in children with Crohn's.

Table 3.2 Typical symptoms of active Crohn's disease determined by disease location

Terminal ileal/ileocaecal	Lower right-sided abdominal pain; diarrhoea; weight loss.
Colonic	Bloody diarrhoea
Small-bowel	Diarrhoea, central abdominal pain; weight loss
Perianal	Pain; discharge; abscesses; skin tags
Oral/gastroduodenal	Upper abdominal pain; indigestion; nausea; vomiting; mouth ulcers; swollen lip.

Crohn's disease has a varied set of symptoms depending on which parts of the gastrointestinal tract are affected. There is often a slow build up of problems, which can take a long time to diagnose as Crohn's disease. Figure 1.4 (Chapter 1) shows the sites commonly affected by Crohn's disease.

Terminal ileal/ileocaecal

This is the commonest site affected by Crohn's disease. This part of the bowel lies in the lower right part of the abdomen. Pain is often felt in this area but may be difficult to localize. If the area affected is quite small, diarrhoea may not be a problem. When diarrhoea does occur it is usually not bloody, as any blood lost is digested by the time it reaches the rectum.

Colonic

Crohn's disease affecting the colon causes symptoms similar to UC. The main symptom tends to be blood-stained diarrhoea. The symptoms will vary depending on how much of the colon is inflamed. Remember that, unlike UC, Crohn's disease can be patchy affecting small or large areas of the bowel with normal areas in between.

Small bowel

Small bowel Crohn's disease normally causes diarrhoea. This tends not to be blood stained. Abdominal pain is another common feature. This may be difficult to localize but is often felt in the middle of the abdomen around the belly button. Other symptoms of small bowel Crohn's disease include weight loss and anaemia.

Perianal

When Crohn's disease affects the area around the anus it can cause a number of symptoms. In addition to fistulas and abscesses (see below) perianal Crohn's disease can cause skin tags. These are small fleshy growths around the anus that are not usually painful but can be irritating. Fissures are breaks in the skin lining the anal canal. These can be very painful when passing stools and may also bleed.

Oral/gastroduodenal

Crohn's disease occasionally causes inflammation in the mouth or upper gut (the oesophagus, stomach, or duodenum). When it affects the mouth it can cause ulceration, which may be painful. It may also cause swelling of the face, particularly the lips. Oral symptoms are mostly found in children and young adults with Crohn's disease (see Chapter 15).

Ulceration in the upper gut may lead to indigestion-like pain, nausea, or vomiting.

Stricturing disease

When the bowel wall gets inflamed in Crohn's disease it can cause narrowing of the gut. This narrowing can become long-standing due to scarring of the bowel wall resulting in a stricture. This can cause a blockage in the bowel. When the flow of bowel contents is obstructed by a blockage in a stricture, it causes pain. If the blockage does not pass quickly the bowel contents will

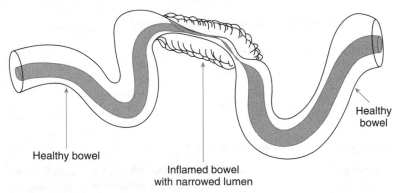

Healthy bowel

Healthy bowel

Inflamed bowel
with narrowed lumen

Figure 3.1 Stricture.

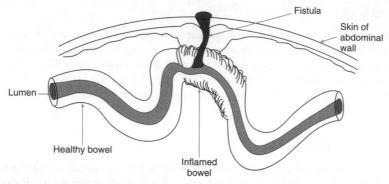

Figure 3.2 Fistula.

build up behind the stricture. This causes severe cramping abdominal pain, nausea, abdominal swelling, and eventually vomiting.

Fistula

Fistulas are caused by inflammation in the bowel creating a break in the bowel wall. This allows a passage to form through to another surface or abdominal organ. The commonest examples are from the rectum to the skin (perianal fistula) or small bowel to skin. Fistulas can leak pus and sometimes bowel contents.

Common types of fistula

- *Perianal*: rectum to skin around anus

- *Enterocutaneous*: small bowel to abdominal wall

- *Rectovaginal*: rectum to vagina

- *Colovesical*: large bowel to bladder

- *Enteroenteric*: bowel to bowel.

Perforation and abscess formation

Perforation occurs when a hole develops in the inflamed bowel wall. Bowel contents can leak through the hole creating a collection of fluid outside the bowel. This will usually form an abscess (collection of pus and infection).

This causes pain and a fever and sometimes a mass. If it is small it may respond to antibiotics but larger abscesses often require drainage. This is normally done by a surgeon or a radiologist.

Abdominal mass

This is a lump that can be felt from the outside of the tummy. It is usually caused by several loops of inflamed small bowel that are stuck together. It is often associated with fistulas, perforation, and abscesses. Abdominal masses are often tender.

Recognizing a relapse of Crohn's disease

As mentioned above, it can be difficult to distinguish between a normal variation in bowel habit and a relapse of Crohn's disease. However, symptoms associated with a relapse include:

◆ diarrhoea

◆ weight loss

◆ pain

◆ bleeding

◆ associated extraintestinal manifestations (see Chapter 13)

◆ new fistula or increase in fistula discharge

◆ fevers.

These symptoms are all suggestive of increasing activity of inflammation. They indicate the need to increase or change treatment. You should therefore contact your doctor.

Conclusions

Inflammation in the gut causes a variety of symptoms depending on which part is affected and how severely. Diarrhoea and abdominal pain are the most frequent problems and are common to both UC and Crohn's disease when active. When IBD is in remission there may be few if any symptoms.

4

General symptoms of inflammatory bowel disease

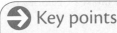 Key points

- People with inflammatory bowel disease can develop a variety of symptoms, such as tiredness and depression, which are not obviously associated with the inflammatory process in their guts.

- These symptoms are very common and can be as troublesome as their gut symptoms.

- Recognizing that they may be caused or exacerbated by inflammatory bowel disease is important.

Introduction

As discussed in Chapter 3, many of the symptoms of inflammatory bowel disease (IBD), such as diarrhoea and abdominal pain, are easily attributable to inflammation of the gut. However, people with IBD may also experience a variety of other symptoms not obviously related to gut inflammation. Nevertheless these symptoms can be equally disabling.

Fatigue

Having active IBD is tiring, both mentally and physically. This is often forgotten by family, friends, colleagues, and employers, perhaps because people with IBD can have no external signs of illness.

There are many potential causes of fatigue in IBD. The first and most obvious is sleep deprivation. The average person requires between 6 and 8 hours sleep a night. Remember, sleep is not just rest, it is a vital process that allows the body and brain to recuperate. As an example, it is thought that sleep is important in the processing of long-term memory. Sleep disturbance is, therefore, potentially very disabling in many ways and can affect our ability to function both physically and mentally.

Getting up at night because of pain or diarrhoea causes sleep disturbance. Even when IBD is inactive the quality of sleep can be impaired. There are theoretical reasons why disturbed nights may contribute to the inflammatory process, although we would not wish to suggest that IBD is caused by lack of sleep!

Fatigue may also be caused by poor nutrition, a common problem in IBD. For example, iron deficiency can cause fatigue. Iron deficiency is common in IBD and can be caused by blood loss (which may not always be visible), or reduced absorption of iron. Inflammation also affects the body's ability to use iron. Fortunately, iron deficiency is relatively easy to identify and also to correct. Other nutritional deficiencies, along with inadequate intake of calories may also contribute to fatigue, as can dehydration (see Chapter 12).

As a final example of why people with IBD can tire easily (although there are many, many more), let's think about active inflammation as a cause of fatigue. Consider how tired even simple viral infections such as colds can make you feel. If you are unlucky enough to have had influenza or glandular fever you will know not only how exhausted these illnesses can make you feel, but also how long tiredness can persist after the infection has passed. The fatigue experienced with viral infections is, in part, related to cytokines, inflammatory chemicals that circulate around the body whenever there is infection or inflammation. In people with IBD, increased amounts of cytokines are also present in the body and can contribute to fatigue.

So, if you're feeling tired and less able to cope with daily living, just think about why that may be. Don't expect too much of yourself and remember it can take a while to recover.

 ## Case study

A 25-year-old woman with ulcerative colitis was admitted to hospital with a flare up that wasn't responding to treatment with oral steroids. She was going to the toilet 10 times per day and getting up twice at night. At home she had two young children and her blood tests showed that she was anaemic. Not surprisingly she also felt exhausted. After a few days in hospital her disease had improved and she received an iron infusion. However, even after discharge, it took her several weeks before she felt her energy levels were back to normal.

Depression

Depression is said to affect about 1 in 10 people at some point. Chronic diseases, such as IBD, can not only make people more vulnerable to depression but can be the sole cause. This is called reactive depression. The unpredictable nature of IBD, along with the severity of its symptoms, means that anxiety and depression are more common in both active disease and remission.

Symptoms of depression

◆ Difficulty sleeping	◆ Excessive tiredness
◆ Loss of sex drive	◆ Loss of appetite
◆ Avoiding social gatherings	◆ Loss of interest in hobbies/pastimes
◆ Feelings of failure/guilt	◆ Feelings of hopelessness
◆ Irritability	◆ Difficulty concentrating

Recognizing depression and dealing with it is extremely important. Antidepressants and/or counselling can be very effective and helpful for some people. Treating depression can also make people better able to deal with the symptoms of IBD. It is even possible that depression could worsen IBD, another reason to take depressive symptoms seriously. Rarely depression can be so severe that people commit suicide. Seeking help sooner rather than later is always better, not least because it is often easier to treat depression in the early stages. Remember, depression is common and is simply another illness. It is certainly nothing to be ashamed of.

Mental function

Many people find that IBD affects their ability to concentrate, study, or work. Of course stress, fatigue, and depression (see above) can all affect how we function mentally, but in IBD other factors can also be important. Iron and other nutritional deficiencies can affect the way our brains work. It is also possible that inflammatory chemicals, such as cytokines (see above) impair our mental function.

Functional gut symptoms

The functional gut disorders are a group of conditions that can cause symptoms similar to those found in people with IBD, such as diarrhoea and abdominal pain. The best known of the functional gut disorders is irritable bowel syndrome (IBS). Unlike in IBD, the bowel looks entirely normal in IBS whether viewed through a colonoscope or under a microscope. The problem is not with inflammation of the gut or with its structure, but rather with its function.

IBS is an extremely common condition and is said to affect up to 1 in 5 (20%) of the population. Indeed, some people with IBD are initially diagnosed with IBS. This is because the two conditions can present in similar ways and IBD, especially Crohn's disease, can sometimes be difficult to diagnose.

It is reasonable to expect that, like the general population, about 1 in 5 people with IBD will also have IBS. However, IBS may be even more common, with some researchers suggesting that up to a third of people with ulcerative colitis and more than half of people with Crohn's disease have functional symptoms. Why should this be so?

A proportion of IBS is brought on by gut infections, so-called post-infectious IBS. It is thought that the initial bowel infection, which causes inflammation, somehow alters the way the bowel works leaving people with altered bowel function after the infection has passed. In some people, this causes IBS. Now, imagine that the bowel inflammation is caused not by an infection but rather by IBD. We know that gut inflammation in IBD is often worse than that caused by infections and is almost always present for much longer. Therefore, if infection can cause IBS, it is easy to understand why IBD may also do so in some people.

Second, we know that there are other triggers for IBS. Like many conditions (including IBD) IBS can be triggered or made worse by stress. For example, think back (or imagine ahead) to when you last took an exam. How many people got abdominal pain or diarrhoea just beforehand? Lots! This is a normal response. The effects of chronic stress, can be very similar. Dealing with IBD itself can, of course, be very stressful and this, in some people, can cause functional gut symptoms.

These are just two examples of why functional gut symptoms may be more common in people with IBD. But why does it matter whether your symptoms are due to active IBD or are functional? Establishing whether symptoms are caused by inflammation or not in IBD can be challenging. If inflammatory symptoms are mistakenly thought to be functional, this can lead to under-treatment. However, if functional symptoms are thought to be inflammatory in origin, unnecessary investigation or treatment can result. In ulcerative colitis, a quick look into the rectum with a sigmoidoscope can often help to sort out this dilemma. Unfortunately, in Crohn's disease the site of inflammation is often less accessible. Although blood tests, radiological examinations, and endoscopies will often provide the answer, these investigations can be time consuming, sometimes uncomfortable and not entirely without risk. Welcome, therefore, to one of the great challenges of managing IBD—perhaps it is no coincidence that the similarly named IBD and IBS are so often confused!

Conclusions

Aside from gastrointestinal symptoms related directly to inflammation in the gut, people with IBD get a variety of less specific symptoms. Recognizing these and their relationship with IBD can be useful as they may require and respond to specific treatment.

5

What tests are performed in people with inflammatory bowel disease?

 Key points

- The tests used to make the diagnosis of inflammatory bowel disease include stool tests, blood tests, X rays, and endoscopic procedures.

- It is normal to require a combination of these tests and many of them are also useful in monitoring the progress of the condition.

Introduction

The diagnoses of Crohn's disease and ulcerative colitis are based on a combination of the symptoms, physical examination, and test results. The tests include simple blood and stool tests, X-rays and scans, and endoscopies. These tests may need to be repeated to reassess the disease.

Blood tests

There are a variety of blood tests that are performed routinely in people being investigated and treated for inflammatory bowel disease (IBD). Several bottles of blood may be required for the different tests although only a tiny volume of blood is taken. Sometimes, blood tests are performed on a weekly basis, for example to monitor treatments. Ward patients may even require bloods on a daily basis. Fortunately, most people will require them much less frequently than this, although yearly blood tests are probably the minimum for someone with IBD.

Table 5.1 Common blood tests

Test	Function
Full blood count	Checks for anaemia and the number of white blood cells
Urea and electrolytes	Checks kidney function and salts. Can show dehydration
Liver function tests	Normally used to look for side-effects of medications. Abnormal in patients with primary sclerosing cholangitis
C-reactive protein (CRP)	A marker of inflammation. Used to monitor disease activity
Erythrocyte sedimentation rate	Another inflammatory marker (ESR)
TPMT	An enzyme involved in the metabolism of azathioprine and mercaptopurine. Often measured prior to starting these drugs.
Iron, B12 and folate	Vitamins and minerals sometimes found to be deficient in IBD

Stool tests

Infections

Everybody gets diarrhoea from time to time. IBD accounts for only a tiny proportion of the diagnoses of people complaining of acute (short-term) diarrhoea. Most such episodes are caused by infections. Of course, people with IBD can get infections too. Therefore, you will normally be asked to provide stool samples to exclude infection when you have active IBD. In studies, about 10% of people with a relapse of IBD are found to have a bowel infection. In some such people, treating the infection improves the diarrhoea and avoids the need to increase treatment for IBD.

Bowel infections are caused by viruses, bacteria, and parasites. Most viral infections are difficult to diagnose and normally improve spontaneously. Stool tests are, therefore, used to exclude bacterial and protozoal infections rather than viral infections. Although a single sample is often enough, sometimes up to three samples are required. Ideally these need to be delivered to the laboratory as soon as possible: the term 'hot, steaming stool' has been used to describe the ideal sample! Of course, this is often practically difficult.

Tests for inflammation

Stool tests that help to distinguish between inflammation and other causes of diarrhoea have recently become available. These detect proteins in the stool produced by white blood cells. They are, however, not routinely available.

Living with inflammatory bowel disease: providing a stool sample

Providing stool samples can be difficult as stool sample pots are normally very small. There are devices that can be put in the bowl of the toilet to help catch a sample, however, these are rarely available in our experience. Perhaps the easiest thing to do (we recognize that even this is not 'easy') is to pass stool into a larger container first (e.g. an old ice cream tub). You can then scoop some into the specimen pot. Some specimen pots have a handy scoop in the lid to help you. If not, an alternative is a disposal plastic spoon.

Radiological tests

The discovery of X-rays by Wilhelm Roentgen in 1895 led to the development of the field of medicine now known as diagnostic imaging. The use of X-rays is, however, only a small branch of this vast and rapidly expanding field and a number of different techniques are commonly used.

Plain X-rays

Plain X-ray films, often seen in the background on medical dramas (normally upside down or back to front!), are a simple snapshot taken of part of the body. For example, they can be used to diagnose fractures because bones show up very clearly. However, they are also used for a variety of reasons in people with IBD. A plain X-ray of the abdomen is the best way of telling if the colon is dilating in patients with severe colitis.

Chest X-rays are also sometimes needed to look for infections or, more rarely, bowel perforation. They are also needed before starting infliximab.

Plain X-rays may also be used to look at the joints in people with IBD-associated arthritis (see Chapter 13).

How barium is used to show us the lining of the gut

◆ *Barium swallow*: the oesophagus is outlined if X-rays are taken as the barium is swallowed.

◆ *Barium meal*: if the X-rays are taken a short time later, the barium has passed into the stomach and duodenum. This allows views of the lining of these parts of the gut.

◆ *Barium follow through*: if, however, the X-rays are taken as the barium leaves the stomach, the small bowel is seen. It can take several hours for the barium to pass all the way through the small bowel

◆ *Barium enema*: barium can be used to visualize the large bowel by infusing the liquid into the colon through a small tube placed in the rectum.

Contrast examinations

The bowel is not particularly well seen with X-rays. However, if it contains a material that shows up well on X-rays, the lining becomes visible. For example, barium, a white chalky substance, can be used to visualize any part of the gastrointestinal tract. Many patients with Crohn's disease will be familiar with barium follow-through examinations. This test is usually not uncomfortable but does take some time (up to 4 hours). Sometimes the radiologist will press on the abdomen while taking a picture to highlight an area of the bowel. A variation of this test is a small bowel enema. For this a small tube is passed through the nose into the first part of the small bowel. This allows larger volumes of contrast to be put into the bowel through the tube to provide better pictures.

Barium enemas, used to image the colon by introducing barium and air through a small tube placed into the rectum, are only rarely used nowadays.

Computed tomography (CT) scans

CT scans are simply lots of X-rays taken simultaneously from various angles. Digitalized reconstruction provides images of cross-sectional 'slices' through the body. The pictures are taken while the patient lies on the machine and automatically moves through an arch. The whole abdomen can be scanned in a matter of seconds. As with contrast X-rays, it is helpful to make the bowel lining stand out. This normally requires drinking some contrast material. Contrast is also injected into a vein, which helps the blood vessels to stand out. The test is painless.

Magnetic resonance imaging (MRI)

Like CT scanning, MRI provides pictures in cross-section through the body. The advantage of MRI is that it involves no radiation relying instead on magnetism to provide images of the body. MRI of the small bowel is a rapidly developing area and is not yet available in some hospitals. As with CT scanning the quality and usefulness of the images obtained is improved by using contrast. MRI is particularly good at imaging perianal fistulas.

MRI scanning takes longer than CT scanning and some people find it more claustrophobic as it involves lying in a tunnel rather than passing through an arch. Nevertheless, most people have no trouble at all. There are some people who cannot have MRIs because of the powerful magnets used to obtain the images. For example, people with pacemakers or certain metal implants cannot have MRIs. You will always be asked about these things before having an examination.

Ultrasound

Anyone who has had a child within the last 30 years will be familiar with ultrasound, which is used to visualize babies in the womb. As the name implies it uses ultrasonic sound waves to produce images of structures inside the body. It involves lying on a table while a probe is pressed on the surface of the body (or rarely placed internally into the rectum or vagina). A jelly-like substance is used to help the sound waves to pass through the skin. It is normally painless although it can be uncomfortable if, for example, the abdomen is tender. This technique is particularly good for looking at organs such as the liver and kidneys or for identifying abscesses. In a few hospitals, it can also be used to look at the bowel. It is completely safe.

Which test and why?

As you can see, there is a huge variety of imaging tests available to help diagnose and manage people with IBD. But how do we know which test to use? There are a several factors that influence this decision. First, not all hospitals provide all tests. Similarly, in some countries governments or private health insurers will not agree to pay for certain tests. Second, some tests are better than others for looking at specific problems; sometimes a plain X-ray may be a better test to do than an MRI. Third, what is good for one person may not be good for another. For example, ultrasound provides better pictures in thin people as there is less distance for the sound waves to travel. Fourth, the choice of imaging technique may be influenced by whether another procedure needs to be performed at the same time. Ultrasound, for example, is sometimes used to help drain an abscess. Finally, there is the issue of radiation. While small amounts of radiation are not harmful, larger amounts are thought to increase the risk of cancers. Therefore, it is important not to use X-rays unless they are necessary. This is particularly important in young people who may be likely to have many tests over the coming years.

Endoscopy

Endoscopes are small flexible tubes that are passed into the body to allow us to see what the lining of the gut (or other body cavities) looks like and to take biopsies. The two forms of endoscopy most commonly performed in people with IBD are gastroscopy (examination of the stomach and duodenum via the mouth) and colonoscopy (examination of the colon and terminal ileum via the anus).

These procedures are normally performed in hospitals. In most hospitals, endoscopy is performed in a dedicated room. Patients often book in at a reception and are then taken through a check-list to confirm their identity and ensure that the correct procedures and preparation have been followed. Depending on the procedure performed, it may be necessary to get changed. A doctor or nurse will ask you to sign a consent form, before taking you in to the endoscopy room. There are normally at least three people in every procedure room, the endoscopist and two assistants, although there may be more. After the procedure you will either be able to leave almost immediately or will return to a recovery area before going home.

Gastroscopy

Gastroscopy is examination of the oesophagus, stomach and duodenum. It is sometimes also referred to as an OGD (oesophago-gastro-duodenoscopy). To ensure the stomach is empty of food and fluid, people fast for at least 4 hours beforehand. The procedure can usually be performed without sedation; an anaesthetic throat spray is used to numb the back of the throat. Some people, however, tolerate the procedure much better if sedated. If possible, you should talk with your doctor about the advantages and disadvantages of sedation before you attend for your procedure.

Gastroscopy takes about 5–10 minutes to perform. Biopsies may be taken and are painless. As with all procedures there are potential risks involved and

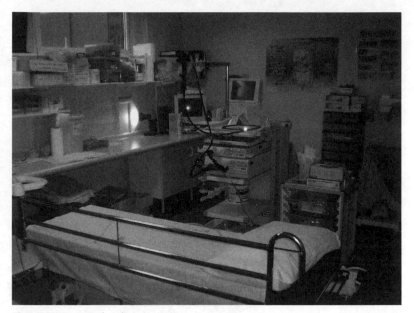

Figure 5.1 A typical endoscopy room.

these will be outlined to you beforehand. In many units, detailed information is sent to people before they attend. The risk of making a hole in the gut with this procedure is said to be tiny, about 1 in 10 000. This can increase if other procedures are performed at the time of the endoscopy, for instance dilating a stricture (narrowing). This would not be performed if it has not been discussed with you prior to the procedure. Other slight risks include aspiration (fluid coming back up from the stomach and going into the lungs) or causing bleeding. Again, these are rare events. If they occur, however, you may need to stay in hospital.

Colonoscopy and flexible sigmoidoscopy

Colonoscopy involves inserting an endoscope through the anus and all the way around the large bowel. It is often possible to insert the endoscope into the last bit of the small bowel, the terminal ileum. In fact, viewing the terminal ileum may be the major reason for doing the test in some circumstances. Because the bowel is normally full of faeces it must be cleared before the test. This involves following a special diet for about 48 hours beforehand. On the day before the test laxatives are used to clear out the bowel.

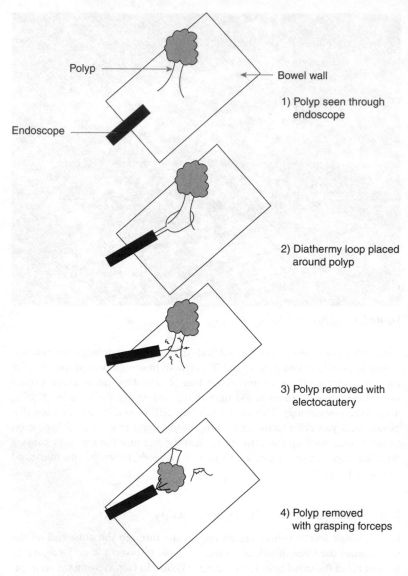

Figure 5.2 Endoscopic polypectomy.

A flexible sigmoidoscopy examines the left side of the large bowel. Even this procedure requires preparation. Some units give the same preparation as for a colonoscopy while others may simply give an enema beforehand. Sometimes, in people with active IBD, flexible sigmoidoscopy or colonoscopy is performed without preparation.

Colonoscopy is normally a simple and straightforward procedure that takes about 20–30 minutes to perform. However, in some individuals it can be more difficult and take longer. It may also take longer if other procedures are performed, such as polypectomy (see Fig. 5.2). The most serious risk of colonoscopy is making a hole in the bowel (perforation). This is said to occur in about 1 in every 1000 procedures. If your bowel is perforated during colonoscopy, an operation is usually needed. If the risks of colonoscopy worry you, talk to your doctor beforehand.

Enteroscopy

The small bowel beyond the duodenum has always been a difficult place to get to with an endoscope. There are, however, extra long endoscopes that are used to look at the small bowel. Until recently, these have always been inserted through the mouth and have been used to view the first metre or so of the small bowel. Recently developed technology has changed this. It is now *theoretically* possible to get to all parts of the small bowel with an endoscope – the upper small bowel via the mouth, and the lower small bowel via the anus. However, this procedure, which requires special equipment and training, is only currently available in a few specialist centres. It is only rarely needed in people with IBD.

Rigid sigmoidoscopy

A rigid sigmoidoscope is a small tube made of plastic or metal that is inserted into the rectum to view the bowel wall. The rectum is gently inflated with air and, if necessary, biopsies can be taken. Unlike the other endoscopy examinations discussed above, this procedure is normally performed in the clinic or on the ward. Because the tube is not flexible, it is not possible to insert it very far. The advantage of the test is that it can be performed immediately rather than requiring a separate appointment.

Capsule endoscopy

In 2000, the first capsule endoscope was swallowed. The procedure is simple. The capsule is the size of a small grape and most people can swallow it easily. A small camera in the capsule beams signals as it passes through the bowel to sensors in a belt worn around the waist. At the end of the procedure (the batteries last for about 8 hours), the images are downloaded and viewed on a computer. The capsule itself is passed out of the body along with the faeces, normally without being noticed. This fascinating new technology does, however, have potential drawbacks. First, because it is new, experience with it is limited. Sometimes, therefore, it is difficult to know exactly what the findings mean. For example, a few small bowel ulcers are seen in many entirely healthy people and their significance is unclear. Fortunately, there is an enormous amount of ongoing research and overall experience of the technology is growing rapidly. The second problem is that capsule endoscopes cannot take biopsies and cannot be steered to have a longer look at an abnormality. The manufacturers of the capsules are, however, working hard on this and other issues. Finally, there is the problem of so-called 'non-natural excretion', or in other words the capsule getting stuck! This can happen if there is a narrowing in the bowel. Therefore, patients with Crohn's disease are at increased risk of this. As surgery is sometimes needed to remove retained capsules, you will be warned of this possibility beforehand and will be asked if you have any symptoms suggestive of a narrowing in the bowel.

Should I have sedation for my procedure?

The answer to this question depends on three things: you, the procedure, and where you have it done. Remember, however, that sedation is not a general anaesthetic. In most centres, you will be awake for the procedure however you have it done. How you react to sedation is very unpredictable and can vary not only from person to person, but also for the same person on different occasions.

What are the advantages of having a procedure without sedation? The most obvious is that once the procedure is over, you can leave immediately and carry on with your day. By contrast, after sedation, you are advised not to drive, sign legal documents, or operate heavy machinery until the following day. Another advantage of unsedated endoscopy is that you can communicate more easily with the endoscopist during and soon after the procedure. The most commonly used sedative in the UK has an amnesic effect, that is, it has a short-acting effect on the memory. This sometimes means that people forget what they are told after their procedure or even, in extreme cases, forget they have had the procedure done!

The procedure

Most people tolerate gastroscopy and flexible sigmoidoscopy without any sedation. In fact, some people tolerate gastroscopy better with throat spray than with sedation. Colonoscopy is normally performed using a mixture of light sedation and a small dose of pain killer. While a few people undergo colonoscopy with no sedation at all, many find this difficult due to discomfort of trapped wind in the bowel. We try to use enough sedation to keep people comfortable but also awake enough to be able to move and speak (many endoscopists ask the patient to move into different positions during the procedure for technical reasons). Safety is also a consideration as oversedation increases the risks of endoscopy.

You

We are all different and while some tolerate procedures better without sedation, others are much more comfortable if they are sedated. If you have any concerns you should discuss them. If possible, you should do so prior to attending for your appointment.

The unit

Some units will routinely sedate all patients for all procedures unless you ask otherwise. More commonly in the UK, however, people are offered the choice of whether to have sedation or not. Practice, however, varies widely from unit to unit and from country to country.

Conclusions

In this chapter, we have covered many of the tests used to diagnose and manage IBD. It is not unusual for the range of tests available to vary from hospital to hospital. This is often particularly the case with newer techniques. It is also important to understand that, depending on the experience and skills of the staff, the best test in one hospital may not be the best test in another. Your medical team will normally recommend that you have the test that they think is going to provide the best information with the minimum of risk and discomfort to you. Sometimes this is clear cut and sometimes it is not. If you aren't sure why you are having a test or want to know if there is an alternative, ask your team.

6

Who looks after people with inflammatory bowel disease?

> ## → Key points
>
> ◆ Inflammatory bowel disease is a complex disease which may require the input of several different health care professionals.
>
> ◆ These include hospital specialists, GPs, nurses, dieticians, psychologists, and counsellors.
>
> ◆ Not all people need input from every member of the team.

Introduction

There will be many professionals involved in your care during the diagnosis and treatment of inflammatory bowel disease (IBD). The approach to care for IBD patients usually (and should) takes the form of a multidisciplinary team.

> ## The multidisciplinary team
>
> ◆ Consultant gastroenterologist
>
> ◆ Consultant surgeon
>
> ◆ General practitioner
>
> ◆ Gastroenterology/surgery registrars
>
> ◆ Ward doctors and nurses
>
> *list continues*

- ◆ IBD nurse specialist

- ◆ Radiologist

- ◆ Pathologist

- ◆ Dietician

- ◆ Psychologist or counsellor

- ◆ Pharmacist

- ◆ Research nurses/fellows.

Which specific members of this team are involved in your care at any particular time depends on whether you are well or unwell, in hospital or at home, needing tests or needing treatment or surgery, or sometimes just needing advice and information.

Role of individual professionals

The section below describes the role of each individual in the order in which you might come across them.

GP

When you first get symptoms of IBD you will probably discuss them with your primary care physician, known in the UK as a GP. The average GP will have only a handful of patients with IBD. As such they cannot be expected to be experts on IBD. Therefore, as soon as they suspect you may have IBD they will want to refer you to your local hospital to see a specialist. This will most likely be a gastroenterologist but might be a surgeon.

Consultant gastroenterologist

This is a doctor who specializes in diseases of the guts. This is usually the person who is responsible for the care of your IBD and normally the leader of the multidisciplinary team. After your diagnosis, you will usually have a named consultant who you should expect to see personally at least once a year. Because IBD is a lifelong condition you are likely to know your specialist for many years and will hopefully build a trusting relationship with them. In larger hospitals two or three consultants may specialize in IBD and work together.

Colorectal surgeon

This is a consultant surgeon who specializes in operations on patients with IBD. Your consultant gastroenterologist will usually work closely with the surgeon and if you are likely to need surgery for your disease your gastroenterologist will refer you to them. Usually the surgical team will take over your care around the time of your operation but will hand back care to your gastroenterology team once you are recovered.

Junior medical team

Each consultant has a team of trainee doctors working with them. This usually includes a registrar or fellow (a qualified doctor training to become a consultant gastroenterologist or surgeon) and ward doctors. In the UK the ward doctors are now known as foundation trainees (previously known as house officers). The team work with their consultant to provide care for you both in the clinic and on the ward.

Consultant radiologist

A radiologist is a doctor who specializes in imaging of the body with X-rays or scans. The gastroenterology team often work with a particular radiologist who will have an interest in bowel disease. The radiologist will advise the team on what scans are likely to help with the diagnosis or assessment of your disease. They will also interpret the images provided by those scans. They may undertake specific procedures, for example, placing a drain into an abscess under X-ray guidance.

Pathologist

The pathologist is a doctor who examines specimens under the microscope. In IBD this usually means looking at biopsies, which are tiny bits of tissue that are removed from the lining of the bowel during endoscopy or colonoscopy. Before the pathologist can examine the biopsies they need to be prepared in a very specific way. This means that the results can take several days to be ready. The pathologist plays a crucial role in securing the diagnosis particularly when there is doubt, for example whether inflammation is caused by ulcerative colitis or Crohn's disease.

Inflammatory bowel disease nurse specialists

The role of the nurse specialist is discussed in more detail in Chapter 7. However, it is worth mentioning here that this person plays a pivotal role in the management of many patients with IBD. It is likely that once you have had IBD for some time you will become very good at recognizing the symptoms and signs of a flare up. What you do when you recognize these symptoms will depend on you, your GP, your IBD nurse specialist, and your gastroenterologist. It is important that you have a plan of what to do in advance rather than having to sort it out at the last minute. In many hospitals, the first point of contact in this situation is the IBD nurse specialist. They will be able to give you advice and to arrange urgent appointments if necessary in the IBD clinic or with your GP.

Psychologist or counsellor

Having something wrong with you is not only unpleasant because of the physical symptoms but is also often a frightening and bewildering experience. It is normal to wonder 'Why me?' Because IBD involves the bowels, many people find it difficult to discuss their symptoms with their close family and friends. A psychologist or counsellor can help you understand your feelings about your disease. They may also be able to help you find ways to overcome some psychological aspects of your illness. Many people feel depressed or angry when they are first diagnosed with a chronic illness. This is particularly likely if you have to have urgent surgery and have not had time to come to terms with your condition. The input of a psychologist or counsellor can be beneficial in these situations. It may also reduce the number of times you visit the doctor or the hospital and may even improve your symptoms.

Some people have specific problems with respect to personal relationships, sexuality, and body image (e.g. coping with a surgical scar or ileostomy). It may be helpful to discuss these with a trained professional.

Pharmacist

In most cases your treatment for IBD will be dispensed either by your local chemist or at the hospital. At the hospital pharmacy there will be a pharmacist responsible for patients with gastroenterological conditions. They will therefore have experience of the particular drugs used for IBD and should be able to answer questions and provide you with information about your drugs. If you have particular concerns about your drugs you should ask to discuss them with the pharmacist when you pick up your prescription.

Some drugs used in IBD require monitoring with regular blood tests. This may be undertaken by the pharmacy, the IBD clinic, by the clinical nurse specialist, or by your GP. The most important thing is that you have your blood tests taken regularly and that someone is checking the results.

Dietician

Because IBD involves the guts, many people are concerned about how their diet affects their disease and their symptoms. The role of diet in IBD is discussed in greater detail in Chapter 12. If you require specific dietary treatment for your IBD you will need to see a dietician. They will go through your normal diet with you and assess your nutritional requirements. During this consultation it may be possible to identify foods that make your symptoms worse. The dietician will be able to advise on healthy eating and why some foods are more likely to make you feel ill. They may also be able to help with weight problems.

The inflammatory bowel disease clinic

Many gastroenterologists, especially those in large hospitals, run clinics specifically for patients with IBD. The benefit for patients is that usually several members of the multidisciplinary team are available in the clinic. Therefore, if you need to see the nurse, as well as the doctor this can easily be arranged.

Because IBD flares up unexpectedly, most IBD clinics have a system that allows you to contact a member of the team urgently when you become ill. This allows urgent appointments to be made for the next clinic rather than having to wait for a routine appointment.

What to expect when you come to clinic

The clinic will usually be run once a week. This will mean that your appointments are likely always to be on the same day. When you attend for an appointment, having booked in with a receptionist and been weighed, you will be called in to see a doctor or nurse (after a variable wait depending on how busy the clinic is!). Because of the number of patients coming to clinic it is not usually possible for the consultant to see every patient every time. The doctor who sees you will be a member of your consultant's team. Even if you have never seen that person before, they should have all your records available to them. Your consultant will usually be in another room in the clinic. If your case is complicated they are always available for their opinion.

If it is your first time at the clinic a detailed history of your symptoms and background will be taken. The doctor will ask you about your recent problems and any previous medical problems, operations, etc. They will also need to know any medications you take. If possible, you should take with you a list of all your medications and the doses you take. You will probably also be asked about your work and any diseases that run in the family.

After taking a history the doctor will usually examine you. The doctor will ask you to lie on a couch. The examination may include looking at your hands, in your mouth, examining your heart and lungs and of course your abdomen.

Finally, it may be necessary and helpful for you to have a rectal examination and rigid sigmoidoscopy. This can be performed while you are lying on the examination couch without special preparation and is done routinely for people with bowel problems especially bleeding.

Having a rectal examination and sigmoidoscopy

You will be asked for your permission to have the examination. A nurse will usually accompany the doctor while they do the examination. If there isn't a nurse there and you would feel more comfortable with someone else being present, then ask. You will be asked to lie down on your left side and remove your lower garments and underwear. You will then bend your knees towards your tummy so that you curl up into a rounded position. The doctor will stand behind you and inspect the area around your anus gently. They will then lubricate the anus with some jelly before inserting a gloved finger gently through the anus into the rectum. This may be slightly uncomfortable and some people find it embarrassing. It shouldn't, however, be painful. A rectal examination allows the doctor to feel for abnormalities in the lower rectum. Once the finger is removed, the glove can be inspected for signs of blood or mucus. Next, the sigmidoscope is inserted through the anus with plenty of jelly. Once the tube is through the anal canal a light is attached to the sigmoidoscope, which allows the doctor to look directly up the tube and view the lining of the rectum. In order to get a good view some air is gently pumped through the tube to inflate the rectum. This will feel like wind in the rectum. Occasionally, a biopsy sample is taken from the rectal lining during rigid sigmoidoscopy by placing forceps through the tube and pinching off a bit of bowel lining. This feels like a little tug but is not painful. The tube is then withdrawn back through the anal canal. You may pass out some of the air that was inserted with it. The whole procedure takes about 2 minutes.

Patients with IBD sometimes need surgery. For this reason in many hospitals the IBD clinic is run jointly between gastroenterologists and surgeons. This allows an on the spot opinion from the surgical team if necessary.

At the end of your consultation you may need some tests. Blood tests are normally done the same day. The results will go back to your consultant in the next day or two. X rays, colonoscopies, and scans usually have to be booked and therefore appointments for these will be sent to you. You will also need to book your next appointment for the clinic with the receptionist.

Most patients with IBD require endoscopies at some point (see Chapter 5). These may not be done by a member of the team looking after you. They are usually done by a gastroenterologist, surgeon, or nurse endoscopist who will let your consultant know the results of the test.

What to expect on the ward

Doctors

The junior members of the team are likely to be the first ones you see if you are admitted to the ward. They will record your details in the hospital notes, arrange tests such as blood tests or X-rays, visit you on a daily basis to check up on your progress and report back to your consultant. Your consultant will usually do a formal ward round with the team twice per week at set times (for example, Dr X does his ward round on Mondays at 9 a.m. and Thursdays at 2 p.m.). You may not be the first patient they see on their round so don't worry if they take some time to get to you; they are very unlikely to have forgotten you! Sometimes your consultant may visit you unexpectedly at other times, for example early in the morning before their clinic. On days when you are not seen by your consultant, you will be seen by the junior members of the team, although you may not be seen at weekends unless there is a specific problem.

Nurses

You will have a nurse in charge of your care on each shift who should introduce themselves to you. At the beginning of your admission a nurse will go through various pieces of information with you. They will take details about you and make sure you are familiar with the layout of the ward, such as where the toilets are and what to do in an emergency. Several times a day a member of the nursing team will come to your bed to take observations. These include your pulse rate, temperature, and blood pressure, although sometimes other things such as your weight and urine output will be checked. The observations are then recorded on a chart, which is normally kept at the end of your bed. You may also be asked to keep a 'stool chart'. This is a record of how frequently you open your bowels. On the chart you write down the time you go, and record whether there was any blood and whether the stool was liquid or solid.

Others

A ward pharmacist will visit at least once during your time on the ward and will go through your medications with you. You will almost certainly meet the phlebotomists who come round every day to do the routine blood tests. You may be collected by porters to take you for tests in different departments. If your doctors and nurses feel it would be helpful, you may also meet other members of the ward team such as the physiotherapist, occupational therapist, dietician, and social worker. Other specialists may be asked to see you while on the ward to give an opinion. If so, you may also see their team as well.

Medical students

Most hospitals, whether they are teaching hospitals or not, provide some teaching for medical students. Medical students normally spend an attachment with a specific team and will attend ward rounds and outpatient clinics. They may also observe operations or investigations (such as endoscopies) and may help out with minor procedures on the ward, such as taking blood or inserting intravenous drips. If you are an inpatient, you may well be asked if you mind if a medical student takes your history and/or examines you. You are not obliged to agree to this. However, seeing patients and learning about specific conditions is vital for all medical students. It also gives you the chance to give them the patient's perspective of having IBD, which is something that they can't learn from books. Without patients seeing medical students, it is impossible to train doctors of the future: all doctors were medical students once. Having said that, if you really don't feel up to seeing a medical student or simply don't want to, you should say so. They will understand.

Most wards have designated visiting times, commonly in the afternoons, when friends and relatives can come to the ward. Visiting outside these times is not generally allowed. This is to allow patients time to rest. It is also easier for the ward staff to do some of their jobs when the ward is relatively empty.

Conclusions

The individual roles of each member of the team should help to make your experience of interacting with the medical service a smooth and supportive one. Because of the complexity of IBD, several specialists may be needed to ensure high quality care and treatment. The multidisciplinary team structure and communication between its members and their patients is crucial to managing IBD.

7

Inflammatory bowel disease nurses

*Della Hughes and Sue Catton IBD Nurses,
Southend University Hospital NHS Trust*

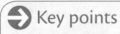 Key points

- Inflammatory bowel disease nurses are a relatively recent concept.

- They fulfil a variety of roles. Some of these overlap with those provided by doctors and some are complementary.

- Some inflammatory bowel disease nurses specialize in more than one area. For example, they may also act as endoscopy nurse specialists or nutrition nurse specialists.

Introduction

Inflammatory bowel disease (IBD) nurses are a relatively new concept. The first IBD nurses were appointed in the UK in the 1990s. Before then, it was recognized that some of the needs of IBD patients were not being met. The introduction of IBD nurses was, therefore, aimed at addressing these issues.

As a result the role of the IBD nurse has evolved rapidly. Roles fulfilled by IBD nurses vary from hospital to hospital depending on local needs. In addition, IBD nurses may act as specialist nurses for more than one specialty and can, therefore, have several groups of patients to support. Despite this variability, IBD nurses aim to provide essentially the same service wherever they are based.

To confuse the issue further, IBD nurses are known by a variety of different titles: some are called Nurse Practitioners while others are known as Clinical Nurse Specialists. Of course, at the end of the day we are all IBD nurses.

The role of the inflammatory bowel disease nurse

Our basic role is to support patients and their families, not only at the time of diagnosis but also through times of trouble. We aim to provide practical expert advice as well as emotional support through the good and the difficult times. The role of the IBD nurse can be divided to cover several different areas (see box below).

Roles fulfilled by inflammatory bowel disease nurses

◆ Providing literature and educational material

◆ Providing emotional support

◆ Running a telephone advice line

◆ Liaising with other doctors, surgeons, or people who may be looking after you

◆ Seeing patients in out-patient clinics, either independently or in combination with doctors

◆ Facilitating rapid access to clinics

◆ Providing in-patient support

◆ Running drug infusion clinics

◆ Managing medication

◆ Immunosuppressant medication follow-up and monitoring

◆ Organizing and/or performing tests, for example, gastroscopy, flexible sigmoidoscopy, and colonoscopy

◆ Co-ordinating colorectal cancer screening in people with IBD

How can an inflammatory bowel disease nurse help

The first time you meet the IBD nurse may be at the time of your diagnosis or soon after. This may be a difficult time for you as you may have many worries and questions. The role of the IBD nurse at this time is to provide you with the information you need to understand your diagnosis and treatment and to help you to come to terms with what your diagnosis means. You may wish to involve other members of your family in discussions as they often have different questions to you. The more they understand the more support they too can offer you. You may be given information in the form of literature from support groups such as the National Association of Colitis and Crohn's Disease (NACC) as well as their contact details and website address. However, the need for information or advice is not just limited to the time of your diagnosis but tends to be ongoing. IBD nurses are available to help with this whether you have just been diagnosed or whether you have had IBD for 30 years. Often the easiest way to get advice is via a telephone helpline.

Telephone advice line

This service varies between hospitals due to the commitments of the IBD nurses. Generally it is a contact number that you can call for advice and information in between appointments. The idea of an advice line is that you always have a point of contact if you are having trouble with your IBD or if you have concerns. Often you will have to leave a message and the nurse will phone you back.

Once you speak to one of the nurses they will either be able to help with your problem over the phone, or if necessary they can arrange for you to be seen in clinic. Alternatively the nurse might liaise with your hospital consultant, general practitioner, or other healthcare professional.

The overall aim is to provide all people with IBD prompt access to advice effective treatment if their disease is flaring up.

 Patient's perspective

Patient surveys show that most people are very satisfied with the service provided by IBD nurses and feel that they are an invaluable member of the team. Here is one patient's views on her IBD nurse:

'When I was first introduced to my IBD nurse I was given her card and was told to contact her if I needed any advice or support. I found it a great relief to know that I could ring and speak to her if I was worried about anything. Over the years, her advice and help along with her words of comfort have been incredibly important to me.'

Out-patient clinics

As many patients are aware when they attend medical out-patient appointments they may see a different person every time. This is because junior doctors tend to rotate between jobs every 6 months or year. The introduction of nurse-led IBD clinics has meant that patients see a familiar face at each visit. Over time the nurse and the patients get to know each other. This can make the consultation a more productive and less worrying experience for some people. A further advantage of nurse-led clinics is that nurses often have more time allocated for each patient. This allows them to spend more time exploring issues that may be of concern.

Drug treatment and monitoring of immunosuppressive medication

Side-effects can occur with any prescribed medication. IBD nurses are very experienced in looking out for and managing these side-effects and can often offer advice about how to minimize them. Similarly, if you are unsure why you are taking a drug or how much you should be taking, your IBD nurse will be able to help clear this up for you.

Many people with IBD take immunosuppressive medication (see Chapter 8). These drugs require regular blood tests to monitor for side-effects. One of the roles that many IBD nurses have taken on is to manage the monitoring of such drugs. Many hospitals have advice sheets regarding immunosuppressive drugs and IBD nurses will be able to provide these and to discuss how the medications may affect you.

Infusion clinics

Increasing numbers of patients with IBD are receiving treatment with biologics (see Chapter 8). One of these, infliximab, is given as an intravenous infusion and this is normally done in hospitals. IBD nurses often organize and run these 'infusion clinics'. Other drugs (such as iron) or blood may also be given at infusion clinics.

Endoscopy

Many IBD nurses are also trained in endoscopic procedures such as gastroscopy, flexible sigmoidoscopy, and colonoscopy. This enables them to be involved in diagnosing IBD and assessing flare ups of disease. For patients, it increases the chance of seeing a familiar face in the endoscopy department.

Colorectal cancer screening

As discussed in Chapter 13, people with ulcerative colitis or colonic Crohn's disease have an increased risk of developing colorectal cancer. To increase the chance of detecting either precancerous changes or early cancers, surveillance colonoscopy is performed in patients at high risk of developing a colonic cancer. Co-ordination of this service is a role that is often taken on by IBD nurses.

Conclusions

Overall the aim of the IBD nurse is to be there for when you need us most, whether you are an in-patient or out-patient. We aim to provide practical advice based on our experience and expert knowledge, often liaising with the medical team who are looking after you. We hope to offer you enough support to make life easier when dealing with IBD.

8

How is inflammatory bowel disease treated?

→ Key points

◆ There is a wide variety of drugs used to treat inflammatory bowel disease and nearly all people with the disease take medication for their condition.

◆ Drugs are used to treat active disease and to prevent relapses occurring when the disease is inactive.

◆ Drugs may also be used to manage symptoms without actually treating the underlying disease.

Introduction

Nearly all people with inflammatory bowel disease (IBD) use medication to manage their condition. The range of drugs available for the treatment of IBD is increasing. Many drugs are used to treat both Crohn's disease and ulcerative colitis, but some are used specifically to treat one condition or the other. The aim of treatment can be split into inducing remission (getting the disease under control) and maintaining remission (keeping it under control).

Route of administration

Drugs for IBD can be given by different routes. These are by mouth (oral), by injection (under the skin, into the muscle, or into a vein), or rectally (inserted through the anus). Some drugs can only be given in one way. For example, infliximab must be given into a vein. Others, however, can be given in several different ways (see Table 8.1). For example, 5-aminosalicylic acids (5-ASAs) can be given either orally or rectally.

Table 8.1 Methods by which drugs are given in IBD

Drug	Oral	Rectal (enema or suppository)	Injection under skin or into muscle	Injection into vein
5-aminosalicylic acids	✓	✓		
Steroids	✓	✓		✓
Antibiotics	✓	✓		✓
Azathioprine/ 6-mercaptopurine	✓			
Methotrexate	✓		✓	
Infliximab				✓
Adalimumab			✓	
Cyclosporine	✓			✓

Ticks indicate routes by which these drugs are normally given to people with IBD.

5-Aminosalicylic acid

5-ASA is commonly used to treat IBD. Its effectiveness in IBD was discovered by chance. Sulfasalazine, a drug containing 5-ASA, was developed to treat patients with inflammatory arthritis. Some patients with IBD who were taking the drug for their arthritis quickly noticed that their IBD was getting better and a new form of drug became available to treat IBD.

Why take 5-aminosalicylic acid?

5-ASA is an effective treatment for mild to moderate ulcerative colitis. It not only treats active disease but, once the disease is under control, 5-ASA also helps to keep the disease in remission. Another possible advantage of 5-ASA in people with IBD is that it may decrease the risk of developing colon cancer (see Chapter 13). Many doctors are, therefore, now encouraging their patients to stay on 5-ASA forever.

5-ASA is also probably effective in some patients with Crohn's disease, although large trials suggest that it is less effective in Crohn's disease than in ulcerative colitis. Nevertheless, as it is safe and well-tolerated, it is often used in people with mild Crohn's disease. 5-ASA may also decrease the risk of colon cancer in people with Crohn's colitis.

5-ASA is sometimes used after surgery to reduce the recurrence of Crohn's disease. It appears to be effective in a minority of patients who have had their small bowel resected.

One disadvantage of 5-ASA drugs is the number of tablets that people have to take. Fortunately, it is often possible to decrease the dose once the disease is controlled. Also, some of the newer forms of the drug need only been taken once a day.

Common 5-aminosalicylic acid-containing drugs in the UK and their trade names

Sulfasalazine: Salazopyrin®

Mesalazine: Asacol®, Ipocol®, Mesren®, Pentasa® Salofalk®

Balsalazide: Colazide®

Olsalazine: Dipentum®

Different forms of 5-aminosalicylic acid

There are several orally administered drugs that contain 5-ASA (see box above). The tablets differ in the way in which they are released in the gut so that some are more appropriate for people with small bowel disease, some for those with colitis, and some for people with distal disease. To explain this better we will briefly explain how the drugs are released.

Sulfasalazine, Balsalazide, and Olsalzine

The active component of sulfasalazine is 5-ASA. This is chemically bound to another compound and until this bond is split, the 5-ASA is inactive. The bond in sulfasalazine needs bacteria to break it down, so the drug is not active until it arrives in the colon where it meets plenty of bacteria. The bond is then broken and the 5-ASA is released. Balsalazide and olsalazine also release 5-ASA in this way. These drugs are, therefore, used to treat inflammation in the large bowel.

Mesalazine

Mesalazine (also known as mesalamine) is 5-ASA by itself. To avoid the drug being inactivated or absorbed before it reaches the desired place of action, manufacturers have devised various delivery systems. One is to put the drug inside a protective coating that will only dissolve at a certain level of acidity (pH). This technology relies on the fact that the pH changes at various points in the bowel. Asacol®, Ipocol®, Mesren MR®, Lialda®, and Salofalk® use this method to deliver the drug to the last part of the small bowel and to the large bowel. A second delivery system is utilized by Pentasa® tablets and granules and Salofalk® granules. These release their contents in a steady stream throughout the gut.

Which 5-aminosalicylic acid should I be taking?

Other than the site of release, the differences between the different formulations of this drug are relatively few; after all, they all contain the same active component. In most countries in the world, sulfasalazine is no longer the drug of first choice as about 20% of people are unable to tolerate it. This is because the 5-ASA is bound to a compound containing sulpha-, which causes allergic reactions or side-effects in some people. However, sulfasalazine is cheaper than the other drugs. For this reason, in some countries it is initially used in all patients to see if they can take it. It is also often used in people who have arthritis and IBD. If you remember the history of the development of sulfasalazine, this should come as no surprise to you.

For some reason, some people get a better response to one form of 5-ASA than another. Therefore, if the 5-ASA you are taking does not appear to be working very well, it may be worth trying a different preparation.

Route of administration

5-ASAs can be taken by mouth or as topical rectal therapy. Enemas or suppositories can be a very effective way of treating inflammation in the rectum because they deliver the drug directly to the site of inflammation. Some people find that they can prevent relapses just by using enemas or suppositories every 2 or 3 days. In more active disease a combination of topical therapy and tablets is often used.

Side-effects

About 20% of patients are unable to tolerate sulfasalazine due to side-effects or an allergic response. Side-effects caused by sulfasalazine include headache, nausea vomiting, and rashes. It can also cause a low sperm count in men (see Chapter 16). This, however, improves when the drug is discontinued.

The other 5-ASA drugs are usually very well tolerated with few side-effects. Rarely but importantly, 5-ASA can actually cause diarrhoea. Other very rare side-effects include inflammation of the pancreas, liver, or kidneys. The only monitoring necessary is a yearly blood test. For sulfasalazine, slightly more regular blood tests are needed.

Living with inflammatory bowel disease: using enemas

People sometimes worry about whether they will be able to use enemas. Most people are perfectly capable of giving themselves enemas. Some people, however, find it easier if they have some help, for instance from their partner (as long as both you and they are comfortable with this). All enemas come with instructions on how to use them, which will differ slightly depending on whether they are liquid or foam enemas. However, some general pointers include:

- Always lubricate the nozzle with some jelly

- Insert the tip gently

- After you have given the enema lie down on your left-hand side. This helps the enema to spread up the colon and increases the chance of you retaining as much as possible of it.

- Try not to go to the toilet soon after giving the enema. However, if you have to go, don't worry too much—you may still have retained some of it.

- Use the enema at night when you are about to go to bed as some people have difficulty retaining enemas when they are upright.

Steroids

Steroids (or corticosteroids) have been used for many years to treat IBD. Steroids are powerful anti-inflammatory drugs. They are not the same as anabolic steroids that are sometimes abused by body builders and sportsmen. They are extremely effective and rapidly improve symptoms in the majority of people with IBD who take them. Unfortunately, they have major drawbacks. For most people they do not keep symptoms under control in the long term and, more importantly, they have potentially serious side-effects. Steroids are, therefore, used in short courses, normally for no longer than 12 weeks.

Route of administration

Steroids can be given as tablets, as injections, or topically into the rectum. Steroids are only given intravenously (into a vein) if oral steroids have failed to work or if the disease is very active. Intravenous steroids are only given in hospital.

Side-effects

The potential short-term side-effects of steroids include weight gain, fluid retention, and increases in appetite and/or blood sugar levels. Rarely, some people find that they get severe psychological disturbances with steroids such as psychosis or depression. Steroid-induced insomnia can usually be prevented by taking them first thing in the morning.

Steroids also increase the chance of developing infections. This is because, like many drugs used to treat IBD, they work by suppressing the immune system. The job of the immune system is to fight infections but, as outlined in Chapter 1, it is also responsible for the inflammation seen in IBD.

Thinning of the bones, which can result in osteoporosis, occurs more frequently in people with IBD (particularly Crohn's disease) than in the general population (see Chapter 13). Steroids can exacerbate this problem. Therefore, calcium and vitamin D supplements are often given to people taking steroids as this may provide a certain amount of protection.

Steroids must be decreased slowly rather than stopped suddenly for two reasons. First, stopping steroids suddenly may increase the risk of a quick relapse. Secondly, and more importantly, steroids are an important hormone produced by our adrenal glands without which we cannot live. Using steroids as a medication for longer than 2–3 weeks suppresses our own natural production from the adrenal glands. If the steroid medication is suddenly stopped the body can be left without any steroid at all. This can be life threatening. Reducing the dose slowly allows the body time to start producing its own steroids again.

Therefore, you should never stop steroids suddenly. It is important to understand clearly how you are going to reduce the dose. It is also important that any doctor, dentist, or nurse you see for any condition is aware that you are taking steroids. You may be given a steroid card by your pharmacist that explains this.

Long-term steroid use is associated with a host of other side-effects, the large majority of which can be avoided if they are used only occasionally for short periods. If steroids are needed frequently, 'steroid-sparing' drugs are required to reduce the risk of long-term side-effects. These are discussed below.

Immunosuppressants (azathioprine, 6-mercaptopurine, and methotrexate)

As their name suggests, these drugs work by suppressing the immune system. They are, therefore, used in people whose disease is poorly controlled by 5-ASAs, or who are requiring recurrent courses of steroids. These drugs are given for long periods of time (years rather than months), and some people will stay on them for life. They are slow acting and may take several months to have their full effects. They are generally used to keep people in remission rather than to induce it.

Route of administration

Azathioprine and 6-mercaptopurine (6-MP) are taken as tablets. Methotrexate is given once a week as a tablet or by injection under the skin or into muscle. For some patients methotrexate works better given as an injection that people can easily learn to do themselves.

Side-effects

Immunosuppressive drugs are generally well tolerated and many people have no adverse reactions at all. Azathioprine and 6-MP are effectively the same drug (azathioprine is converted to 6-MP in the body). Serious side-effects include suppression of the white blood cell count, liver abnormalities, and pancreatitis. In fact, the white blood cell count drops slightly in most people taking azathioprine or 6-MP without causing any problems. However, in some people the white blood cell count can drop to dangerously low levels. This leaves the body unable to fight infections properly and can therefore be dangerous. Azathioprine and 6-MP can also cause inflammation of the liver (which does not normally cause symptoms in the early stages). Pancreatitis (inflammation of the pancreas) may rarely occur and causes severe pain in the upper abdomen. Fortunately, all these side-effects improve when the drug is stopped. However, if severe they may require admission to hospital. Methotrexate can also cause suppression of the white cell count and liver abnormalities.

During the first few weeks of treatment regular blood tests are needed. This means that if one of the more serious side-effects does occur it is detected early. In particular, regular liver tests and white blood cell counts are performed. There is also now a test (TPMT) available in most parts of the world that will predict the 1 in 300 people who will, for genetic reasons, predictably react very badly to azathioprine and 6-MP. Once treatment is stabilized, blood tests are necessary every few months to monitor for side-effects.

Less serious side-effects include nausea, headaches, and flu-like symptoms, which frequently improve after the first few weeks of treatment. About half of people who are unable to tolerate azathioprine are able to take 6-MP instead. All people taking methotrexate should be on folic acid tablets too which reduces many of the milder side-effects.

There is concern that immunosuppressant drugs increase the risk of developing lymphoma, a rare form of cancer of the lymph glands. However, people with IBD, particularly those with very active disease, may be at a slightly increased risk of getting lymphoma anyway (see Chapter 13). Of course, people with very active disease are the ones who are treated with immunosuppressants. It has therefore been difficult to establish whether the slight increase in lymphoma is related to drug, disease, or both. Nevertheless, the latest research suggests that there is about a fourfold increase in risk of developing a lymphoma associated with taking azathioprine or 6-MP. To put this in perspective, the risk for people age 20–40 is increased from approximately 1 in 10 000 per year to 4 in 10 000 per year (both of which are very small). It is important to weigh up this risk against the alternatives. These may include using other drugs such as steroids (which have their own risks), leaving the disease untreated, or undergoing surgery. The risk of azathioprine-induced lymphoma increases with age such that people in their 70s have about a 1 in 1000 background risk per year of developing lymphoma.

Azathioprine and 6-MP also slightly increase the risk of developing some forms of skin cancer. It is, therefore, particularly important for people who take these drugs to use sunblock and to limit their sun exposure.

Methotrexate can cause lung damage. However, this may occur less frequently in people taking methotrexate for IBD than when they take it for other conditions. If you are taking methotrexate and become short of breath, you should let your doctor know.

Cyclosporine

Cyclosporine is another powerful immunosuppressant. It is sometimes given to people with very severe ulcerative colitis whose disease is not responding to intravenous steroids. It is used in an attempt to avoid an operation and is successful in the short term in about 70% of people who receive it. Unfortunately, cyclosporine also increases the risk of infection and has several other side-effects. These include kidney damage, high blood pressure, and, rarely, seizures. At the dose used in ulcerative colitis, serious side-effects are unusual. Cyclosporine is not used as long-term maintenance for ulcerative colitis. Instead, an alternative immunosuppressant is started allowing the cyclosporine to be discontinued after a few months.

Route of administration

Cyclosporine is usually given intravenously as a continuous infusion when it is used in acute severe colitis. It can, however, be given orally but some people worry that this may be less effective. If it works, the infusion is swapped for oral capsules of cyclosporine after a few days. These can be continued after discharge, although regular monitoring in the clinic and blood tests for drug levels are needed.

 Case study

A 26-year-old man was admitted to hospital after he presented to the emergency department with a 3-week history of bloody diarrhoea. The diagnosis of ulcerative colitis had only been made 6 months previously and this was his first flare up since. Despite starting treatment with intravenous steroids he was still opening his bowels frequently with no improvement in his symptoms after 3 days.

He had consultations with his Consultant Gastroenterologist and a Consultant Colorectal Surgeon at which the options of infliximab, cyclosporine, and surgery were discussed. Between the three of them they agreed to try treatment with cyclosporine. Fortunately, he responded quickly to this and was able to go home 10 days later.

Biologics (infliximab and adalimumab)

These drugs have become available over the last 10 years. They interfere with specific steps in the inflammatory response. Infliximab (Remicade®) was the first biologic to be used in IBD, initially only in people with Crohn's disease. Recently, however, it has also been shown to be effective in ulcerative colitis and has even been used in people with very severe colitis as an alternative to cyclosporine. Trials are currently underway to discover which is the better and/or safer of these drugs to use in this situation. If your doctor is considering treating you with these drugs they will have an in-depth discussion with you about the relative merits of each of them compared with surgery.

Adalimumab (Humira®) is a similar drug to infliximab and is used for Crohn's disease. Several other biologics are currently undergoing trials and are likely to become available over the coming years. The biggest drawback of these drugs is their cost. Because of this, their availability is limited in some parts of the world. However, competition will probably drive their cost down in the future.

Route of administration

Infliximab is given as an intravenous infusion, normally in hospital. If used to maintain remission it is given every 8 weeks. Adalimumab is given by subcutaneous injection every other week. With simple training people can learn to do this by themselves at home.

Side-effects

These drugs like, steroids and immunosuppressants, can make people more likely to get infections. Of particular concern is the risk of getting or reactivating tuberculosis (TB). Therefore, before starting biologic drugs, tests are done to identify people at high risk of TB. These tests vary from hospital to hospital and country to country because of the ethnic make up of the local population and the background rates of TB. A chest X-ray is nearly always performed and specific blood or skin tests may also be done. If evidence of inactive TB is found, or if people have recently moved from areas where TB is common anti-TB treatment may be needed. Active TB is always treated before using infliximab or adalimumab. Some doctors also advise that certain foods, such as cheeses made from unpasteurized milk, should be avoided to decrease the chance of exposure to a bacterium called *Listeria*.

The risk of lymphoma with biologics is unknown, but may be slightly increased. Again it is important to remember that the risks of serious side-effects from these drugs is low and the potential benefits are high. About a million people have received infliximab worldwide and very few have had serious problems related to the drug.

Nutritional therapy

General aspects of diet and nutrition are extremely important and are covered in their own chapter (Chapter 12). People with IBD often wonder if their disease can be treated by altering their diet. Indeed, it is actually possible to treat small bowel Crohn's disease with nutritional therapy. In fact, in children, this is often used as the first line of treatment. This is because it avoids the need to use steroids that can affect growth, and because children with Crohn's disease are often undernourished. The treatment, known as an elemental or polymeric diet, uses a drink that provides all nutritional requirements. The drinks are made up of the basic components of food (see Chapter 12) and during the treatment, no normal food is eaten. Unfortunately, because the drinks do not taste very nice and because no other food is allowed some people do not like nutritional therapy. Because of the taste, many people on nutritional therapy prefer to be fed at night through a nasogastric tube (a tube passed through the nose into the stomach). This can be done at home and many children and some adults with Crohn's disease use this form of treatment. A typical course lasts 6–8 weeks.

Whether nutritional therapy can keep Crohn's disease in remission or not is less clear and, unfortunately, the disease often relapses once a normal diet is resumed. Of course, if you remember that nutritional therapy seems to work best when all other food is excluded it becomes apparent why it is not a popular treatment with adults, particularly in the long term.

Antibiotics

Antibiotics, such as ciprofloxacin and metronidazole, are sometimes used to treat active Crohn's disease. However, trials suggest that they are only marginally effective, if at all. Nevertheless these drugs are well tolerated with few serious side-effects and are therefore sometimes used as an alternative to steroids in people with mild Crohn's disease.

Where antibiotics are definitely useful is as a treatment for infections. In people with fistulas, they can decrease drainage from the fistulas and treat abscesses. Metronidazole and other drugs like it can also decrease the risk of recurrence after operations for Crohn's disease. However, treatment must be taken for several months and is sometimes limited by side-effects.

Route of administration

Antibiotics are normally taken as tablets. Both metronidazole and ciprofloxacin can be given intravenously and metronidazole can also be taken as a suppository.

Side-effects

Ciprofloxacin is very well tolerated by most people. A common side-effect of metronidazole is to make people nauseated. It can also cause mild nerve damage in the fingers and toes if taken for long periods.

Other drugs: symptomatic treatment

Many other drugs are used by people with IBD not as a treatment for the condition itself but rather to help control the symptoms.

Loperamide and codeine phosphate are drugs used to treat diarrhoea. They can be very helpful, particularly for people with pouches (see Chapter 9) or short bowel syndrome (see Chapter 13). However, their use is discouraged in people with acute attacks of colitis. This is for two reasons: first, because they can falsely mask symptoms of active disease and second, because they can increase the risk of developing a dilated colon. Dilatation of the bowel, also known as toxic megacolon is a life threatening condition and requires surgery before the bowel perforates (see Chapter 9).

Abdominal pain is a common symptom in IBD and arthritis affects about 1 in 5 people with IBD. **Pain-killing drugs** are therefore sometimes necessary. **Paracetamol** does not normally cause any problems in people with IBD. **Non-steroidal anti-inflammatory drugs (NSAIDs)**, such as **ibuprofen** and **diclofenac**, are extremely effective pain killers, particularly for people with joint pain. Unfortunately, they can cause IBD to flare up and are generally avoided if possible. **Opioid painkillers** such as **codeine**, **pethidine**, and **morphine** are also very effective painkillers. As mentioned above their use in acute severe colitis is avoided because of the risks of colonic dilatation.

Often, pain and diarrhoea are signs of active disease and, while pain killers and antidiarrhoeal drugs can help with symptoms, treatment of the underlying IBD is what is really needed.

Nutritional supplements such as **iron** and **folic acid** are covered in Chapter 12.

Which drug and when?

There are, of course, whole textbooks written about how to treat IBD and there is often no single correct answer as to which drug should be used at any particular time. The decision needs to be made jointly by the person with IBD and their team of health professionals.

Principles of drug treatment

The first aim of treatment is to get the disease under control, that is, in remission. Depending on the severity of the disease this may require the use of 5-ASA, steroids, nutritional therapy, and/or biologics. Once the disease is in remission, drugs can help to prevent relapse. Steroids are not appropriate for this. 5-ASA can help prevent relapses as can biologics, and immunosuppressants are also used for this purpose.

In general, mild disease can often be managed without having to use immunosuppressants and biologics and sometimes it can be appropriate for

Table 8.2 Remission and maintenance agents

Drugs used to get disease into remission	Maintenance agents
5-aminosalicylic acids	5-aminosalicylic acids (UC)
Steroids	6-mercaptopurine/azathioprine
Antibiotics (?) (CD)	Methotrexate (mostly CD)
Nutritional therapy (CD)	Nutritional therapy (?) (CD)
Infliximab	Infliximab
Adalimumab (CD)	Adalimumab (CD)

CD, Crohn's disease; UC, ulcerative colitis.

people to be on no treatment at all. The standard practice is to use treatments sequentially starting with 5-ASA, working up through steroids and immunosuppressants. In general, biological agents are reserved for those who fail to respond to the other treatments. Currently, there is a considerable amount of research investigating whether we should reconsider our approach to the management of IBD. For example, it may be that in the future, we use the most powerful agents much earlier in an attempt to get the disease under control sooner. The disadvantage of this approach is that it would mean exposing a lot of people to the potentially serious side-effects of these drugs when many of them may not have needed the drugs at all.

Drug interactions

One of the reasons that it is important to know which drugs you are taking is to minimize the chance of drug interactions. Doctors and pharmacists always ask what drugs you are already taking before providing you with new medication. The safest thing to do is probably to have a list of your medication and doses that you can carry on your person.

Many drugs interact with each other. While many interactions are unimportant some interactions may make one of the drugs work less well while others may make one of the drugs overly active, potentially causing side-effects. Drug interactions can also occur with medications that you can buy over the counter. As an example, methotrexate can have a potentially serious interaction with aspirin and NSAIDs. Some medications interact not only with other drugs but also with some foodstuffs. Cyclosporine, for example, can interact with grapefruit juice.

Conclusions

As you can see, a wide variety of drugs are used to treat IBD. In this chapter we have discussed the most commonly used. Most people with IBD will be on a variety of drugs throughout the course of their lives. Often more drugs are needed when the disease is active and fewer when it is inactive. It is important that you should know why you are taking each drug and what side-effects you may get. You should also know what monitoring is required for your treatment. As always—if you are unsure about any of this, ask.

9

Surgery for inflammatory bowel disease

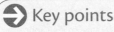 Key points

- Many people with inflammatory bowel disease require surgery at some point.

- Which operation is required depends on whether the underlying diagnosis is ulcerative colitis or Crohn's disease, where the disease affects, and what sort of problem it is causing.

- The commonest operations are colectomy, with or without pouch reconstruction, right hemicolectomy, small bowel resection, and stricturoplasty. Some operations can now be done by keyhole surgery.

Approximately 70% of people with Crohn's disease and 30% of people with ulcerative colitis require surgery for their condition at some point. The sort of surgery required depends on both the problem and the underlying condition.

Reasons for surgery

Ideally, surgery is performed electively. In other words, the surgery is planned and discussed in advance, the patient is admitted to hospital shortly before the operation and the surgery is performed on a predetermined date. However, sometimes surgery needs to be performed urgently (in other words within a few days) or as an emergency (within a few hours). Urgent or emergent operations are performed because delaying them would potentially endanger the patient's health or even threaten their life. For example, a perforation of the bowel in a patient with severe ulcerative colitis needs emergency surgery as

Table 9.1 Common operations in inflammatory bowel disease

Name	Description	Disease
Total colectomy	Removal of entire colon	Ulcerative colitis, Crohn's disease
Right hemicolectomy/ ileocaecal resection	Removal of terminal ileum and part of right colon	Crohn's disease
Small bowel resection	Removal of segment of small bowel	Crohn's disease
Stricturoplasty	Opening up area of narrowed bowel	Crohn's disease
Ileostomy	Formation of an opening of the small bowel on to the abdominal wall	Ulcerative colitis, Crohn's disease
Reconstruction surgery/ pouch formation	Various ways of joining the bowel together to make a continuous tube to the anus	Ulcerative colitis, Crohn's disease
Perianal abscess drainage and seton placement	Drainage of abscess. Placing a string (seton) through a fistula to prevent abscess formation	Crohn's disease

Table 9.2 Indications for surgery

Emergency	Perforation of bowel
	Uncontrollable bleeding
Urgent	Deterioration of acute severe colitis despite intensive drug therapy
	Dilatation (expansion) of colon suggesting imminent perforation in severe colitis
	Small bowel obstruction or inflammation not responding to intensive drug therapy
	Intra-abdominal or perianal abscess not responding to antibiotics
Elective/planned	Colonic or ileocolonic stricture
	Chronic active colitis despite treatment
	Dysplasia or cancer
	Fistula causing symptoms

leaving it untreated is life threatening. Table 9.2 summarizes the situations in which emergency, urgent, and elective operations are performed.

Ulcerative colitis

The commonest reason for needing surgery in ulcerative colitis is when drug treatment fails to control symptoms. This occurs in two different circumstances. The first is in a severe flare of colitis when decisions have to be taken quickly (day by day) to prevent deterioration or perforation of the colon. In this scenario the person will be in hospital and their response to drug treatment will be being monitored very closely. Monitoring includes the recording of stool frequency, rectal bleeding, pulse rate, blood pressure and temperature, and also performing daily blood tests. Thankfully, it is extremely rare for the colon to perforate. However, to avoid this and other complications of severe colitis an operation is often considered. It is actually required in about 10% of all severe colitis episodes.

The second situation is when increasing medication fails to control colitis so that the person is chronically unwell. Often they will have put up with poorly controlled symptoms for months despite many clinic visits and several different treatments. In this case the operation can be booked in advance (elective surgery). Some of the preparation for surgery is done in outpatients and, therefore, admission to hospital may be on the day of the surgery.

People with colitis who have been found to have dysplasia (precancerous changes) or cancer, will also have elective surgery.

Colectomy for acute severe colitis

This describes an urgent procedure done during admission to hospital for acute severe ulcerative colitis.

Normally you will have been in hospital for a few days having treatment with intravenous steroids, but without responding fully. The medical and surgical teams will explain carefully the risks of continuing with steroids, trying an alternative drug or having surgery. Usually a date is set for surgery (e.g. a few days ahead). If your condition has not improved adequately by this time, then surgery goes ahead. Ideally these operations are performed on a weekday when the consultant colorectal surgeon is there to do your operation. As well as meeting your surgeon and their team before an operation, you will also be introduced to the stoma nurse. He/she will explain what a stoma is and how it works and will discuss the best site for it.

Emergency colectomy is performed when the bowel perforates or bleeds uncontrollably. In this situation you may only meet your surgeon shortly before going to theatre and you may not have the chance to talk to a stoma nurse as delaying surgery may be life threatening.

(See also Chapter 8—case study)

Having an operation

All operations will follow some but not necessarily all of the following process. If you are not in hospital already, you will be admitted shortly before the planned operation date. You may be asked to take bowel preparation (as for colonoscopy), although this may not be necessary if your colitis is active. You will be starved for several hours before the operation. The ward staff will ask you to change into a theatre gown (a sort of nightdress) and will go through a checklist with you (such as checking that you have removed your jewellery and whether you have any false teeth). An anaesthetist may visit you on the ward before you go to theatre. This is the doctor who will put you to sleep for your operation. They will check your medical history and explain the anaesthetic to you. They may also discuss the options for pain relief after the operation.

You will be wheeled to the operating theatres on a trolley accompanied by one of the ward nurses. Before you go into the operating theatre, you will be taken into a brightly lit room called the anaesthetic room where you will be given the anaesthetic. An anaesthetic involves breathing oxygen through a mask held over your face while you are given an intravenous injection to make you unconscious. When you are fully asleep a tube is placed into your throat to allow a machine to control your breathing. You will be transferred into theatre and on to an operating table where your surgeon will be waiting.

Afterwards you will be taken from the operating theatre to the recovery area where you will start to come round from the anaesthetic. Gradually you will become aware of your surroundings and of people talking to you. The anaesthetist will have set up an infusion of painkillers and antisickness drugs. The dose of these can be adjusted to keep you comfortable. Often there will be a button you can press to give a dose of painkiller when you start to feel any pain. This is called patient-controlled anaesthesia (PCA) and you will have this the first day or two back on the ward.

When the theatre staff are happy you are awake enough you will be wheeled back to the ward. This may be a different ward to the one you came from. Some patients may spend some time on the intensive care unit or high dependency unit after surgery. Most people, however, will go back to a normal surgical ward. You will probably have at least one drip infusing fluids and drugs into your veins and a catheter tube in your bladder to drain urine into a bag. These are not permanent but will help you recover more comfortably. If you have an ileostomy it will be covered by a bag. The nurses and surgeons will inspect your stoma to check it is healthy.

The surgical team will usually visit later in the day or the next morning to see how you are recovering from your operation. As you feel better you will be allowed to sip water, then drink to fluids, and finally to eat.

Meanwhile, if you have a stoma, your stoma nurse will also visit regularly to check the stoma, and to help you understand how it works and what to do with it. The medical gastroenterology team may also visit you and advise on reducing your medications as you get better.

Over the next few days you should feel stronger and healthier. You will be encouraged to get out of bed and to walk to the toilet. When you, your surgeons, your stoma nurse, ward nurses and physiotherapists are all happy you are ready, you will be discharged home. An appointment will be made for you in the surgical outpatients a few weeks later to come back for a check up. At that time you will have the chance to discuss any future surgical options (see below).

Reconstructions after colectomy

Two- and three-stage pouch surgery

After a colectomy, a further operation can be performed at which the end loops of the small intestine can be sewn together to form a bag known as a pouch (see Fig. 9.1). This is then attached to the anus and acts like a new rectum, storing faeces. The pouch is left to heal for several weeks by the formation of another ileostomy, usually at the same site as the previous one. At a third operation 2–3 months later the ileostomy is closed and the small bowel is reconnected to the pouch to allow faeces to pass directly through to the anus. Sometimes when people have an elective colectomy, this whole process is performed in two rather than three operations. Pouch surgery is not normally performed on patients with Crohn's disease as the condition almost always recurs in the pouch.

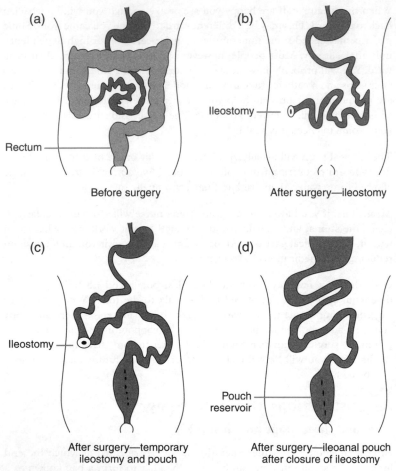

Figure 9.1 Three-stage proctocolectomy and ileoanal pouch formation.

Ileorectal anastomosis

Less commonly the rectum is left in place and the small bowel is joined directly on to it. This is called an ileorectal anastomosis. Because the rectum is still present a pouch is not necessary. However, it is still possible for disease to recur in the rectum, which may, therefore, require regular examinations to check for recurrent disease or dysplasia.

Bowel function after ileoanal pouch surgery

Bowel function following pouch surgery varies. Because the colon and rectum have been removed, stool that comes through the pouch to the anal canal is liquid. This means that stool frequency is increased. The average stool frequency over 24 hours is about four to six bowel motions. People with pouches often take antidiarrhoeal drugs such as Imodium, to reduce stool frequency. Many people who have had pouch surgery also get urgency and find that they cannot hold on very long after the first sensation of desire to open the bowels. This also means that they may have to get up at night to pass faeces. For this reason it is important to have good anal sphincter strength prior to pouch surgery. Patients who have a weak anal sphincter may be advised against a pouch because of the risk of leakage and incontinence. Urgency and nocturnal defecation seem to improve with time as the pouch matures. Overall about 15% of patients who have had surgery may end up with further complications and some have to have their pouch removed leaving them with a permanent ileostomy. However, the majority of patients go on to have a very good quality of life after pouch surgery.

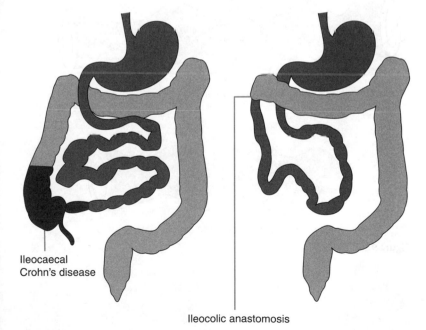

Ileocaecal
Crohn's disease

Ileocolic anastomosis

Figure 9.2 Right hemicolectomy.

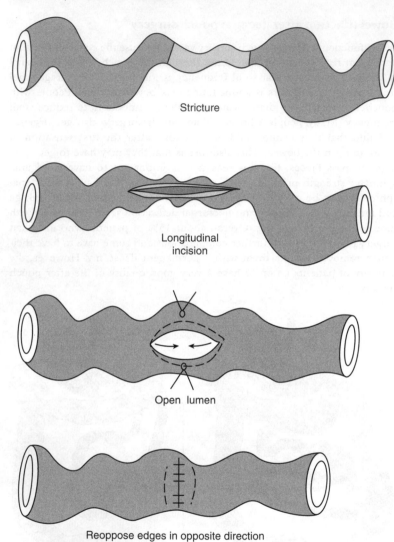

Stricture

Longitudinal
incision

Open lumen

Reoppose edges in opposite direction

Figure 9.3 Stricturoplasty.

Right hemicolectomy

This is done to remove Crohn's disease affecting the terminal ileum and caecum. The healthy end of the remaining ileum is joined directly on to the colon.

Small bowel resection

This describes an operation to remove a segment of small bowel that is inflamed, strictured, or fistulating. The entire disease segment is cut out and the two remaining healthy ends are joined back together.

Stricturoplasty

This operation was invented as a way of opening up narrowing in the bowel without having to cut out whole sections. If there are several strictures this reduces the risk of the remaining bowel being left too short to carry out its normal function.

As shown in the diagram the narrowed segment of bowel is opened along its length in a slit. This is then sewn back together in the horizontal plane. This opens the internal narrowing to relieve the blockage but only minimally shortens the segment of bowel. This can be a very effective way of treating strictures. However, because the disease has not been entirely removed, the strictures are prone to recur.

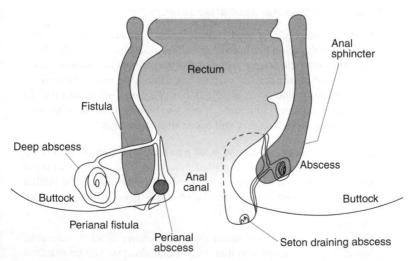

Figure 9.4 Perianal fistula.

Drainage of perianal sepsis

When abscesses and fistulae develop in the perianal area they can form a complex network of collections of infection linked together by tracks within the tissues. These are painful and distressing and can form large abscesses if not treated appropriately. MRI scanning is often used to get a clear picture of the anatomy of the fistulae. However, the alternative is for the surgeons to examine the area with the patient under anaesthetic. You may hear this being called an EUA (examination under anaesthetic). During the procedure, the surgeons will carefully examine the perianal area for the opening of fistulae. They can also examine internally for openings. They can use small curetting instruments to open up fistulae and to let pus and infection drain out. They may also insert a seton. Setons may be a small thread, or a larger rubber tube through the fistula into the abscess cavity. The seton is tied so that it forms a loop between the internal opening of the fistula (i.e. inside the rectum) and the external opening on the perianal skin. This means that any remaining pus can more easily drain out along the track formed by the seton. This helps to prevent further formation of abscesses.

Fistulas will not heal satisfactorily when there is ongoing infection. Setons are, therefore, often left in place for weeks or months before being removed. Removal can usually be done easily without the need for an anaesthetic.

❓ Frequently asked questions

Will the disease come back after surgery?

◆ *Ulcerative colitis:* after a total colectomy for ulcerative colitis, the vast majority of the colon has been removed. As ulcerative colitis only affects the large bowel the disease cannot come back. There is, however, sometimes a few centimetres of rectum left behind for technical reasons. If this rectal stump (as it is called) causes a lot of symptoms due to continuing or recurrent disease, it can also be removed. Some extraintestinal manifestations may still occur after colectomy.

In addition, some patients who have had pouch operations develop inflammation in the pouch, called pouchitis. This causes increased stool frequency and occasionally bleeding. It can usually be settled down with antibiotics. Fortunately, pouchitis is not usually as severe as the previous ulcerative colitis.

◆ *Crohn's disease:* if the operation does not remove all of the diseased bowel (e.g. stricturoplasty) then ongoing medication will be required to treat the remaining areas of affected bowel and to try to prevent the need for further surgery.

Even if all the affected bowel is removed during an operation, the risk of recurrence of disease is very high. However, recurrent Crohn's disease can often be controlled with medication. As an example, 50% of people who have had their terminal ileum and caecum removed (probably the most commonly performed resection for Crohn's disease) will not need further surgery within the next 10 years.

The risk of recurrence can be reduced by using medication. After your operation your gastroenterologist will discuss with you which drugs would be the most suitable for you to use. There is often more than one option (including taking no treatment at all) and you will be able to discuss the risks and benefits of each of the options.

- *Smoking:* if you are a smoker, the most effective way of preventing recurrence of Crohn's disease after an operation is to give up smoking. This is more effective than any drug.

 Case studies

Although people are normally keen to avoid surgery, many people with inflammatory bowel disease feel so much better after surgery that they wished they had had it done sooner. Here are two patients' experiences of surgery.

Kathy* was a 47-year-old publican who had been diagnosed with ulcerative colitis a year ago. Since diagnosis she had required several courses of steroids and had taken azathioprine for the previous 6 months. Although her symptoms were variable she had never gone into complete remission and eventually came into hospital for intravenous steroids. Although this improved her symptoms slightly, she was still going to the toilet five times a day and was regularly passing blood. More to the point, she felt exhausted, had no appetite and was therefore losing weight. After several discussions about her options with her gastroenterologist and colorectal surgeon she decided to have a colectomy. She recovered from the operation very quickly and was back to work within a few weeks. She was able to stop all her treatment and regained her energy rapidly. She felt so well that she decided that she wished to keep her ileostomy rather than undergo further surgery.

David* was 22 when he was admitted to hospital with severe cramping abdominal pain. Investigations showed that he had Crohn's disease affecting the last 10 cm of his ileum. His symptoms settled down on steroids and he was discharged home. Over the coming months he continued to get episodes of severe pain. Surgery was discussed but David was worried about taking time off work. Despite treatment his pain continued and he ended up having to take more and more time off work. He was also losing weight and feeling increasingly tired. At this point David decided to have an operation. He had keyhole surgery to remove the diseased section of bowel and was out of hospital in a few days. Five years later he remains asymptomatic and is not taking any treatment, perhaps partly because he gave up smoking at the time of his operation.

*Names changed

Larger abscesses are drained in a similar way, sometimes with a sort of wick left in the depths of the cavity coming out on to the skin to allow continuing drainage of pus.

Keyhole surgery

Recent advances in surgical techniques mean that some operations can now be done by keyhole surgery, also known as laparoscopic surgery. These operations have smaller scars and often have shorter recovery times. However, not all surgeons practise this form of surgery.

Conclusions

Most people with Crohn's disease require surgery at some point in their lives. The operation performed depends both on the site and the nature of the disease. Although disease is likely to recur at some point, surgery can produce long periods of good quality of life in between.

For ulcerative colitis, a colectomy is needed in about a quarter of cases. Reconstructive surgery (pouch formation) is often possible after colectomy for ulcerative colitis.

10

Complementary and alternative medicine in inflammatory bowel disease

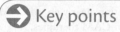
Key points

◆ Complementary and alternative therapies are frequently used by people with inflammatory bowel disease.

◆ Although there are limited clinical trial data available to support their use, many people perceive benefits from them.

◆ A small number of trials have shown that some sorts of complementary and alternative medicine are effective in inflammatory bowel disease.

◆ Complementary and alternative medicine, like all medicine, can have side-effects and can interact with conventional medicine.

Complementary and alternative medicine

Complementary and alternative medicine (CAM) is exactly what it says it is. In other words, it describes medical theories and practices that are complementary or alternative to conventional medicine. The combined term, CAM, includes a vast and varied range of procedures and concepts of health and disease. These include traditional practices such as acupuncture, traditional Chinese medicine, Ayurvedic medicine, homeopathy, and herbal medicine, as well as more modern complementary practices, including aromatherapy and reflexology.

Because most types of CAM are outside the area of conventional scientific medicine, there has been very little high quality research conducted on them. Similarly, CAM tends not to be taught at medical school. Alternative medicine practices are often based on ideas or beliefs that ignore modern science. Instead they rely more on ancient practices and 'natural' remedies. These are often thought of as being less toxic than conventional drugs. This, of course, makes them attractive to many people, especially those suffering with chronic disease that have not responded well to conventional treatment.

However, most information relating to the possible effectiveness of CAM is anecdotal or historical. This compares with most conventional medicines that have been through rigorous scientific trials to prove that they work and are safe (see Chapter 11). Therefore, many doctors and healthcare professionals are sceptical about CAM. This attitude is definitely changing across the world. In inflammatory bowel disease (IBD) there is an increasing awareness and a desire to apply clinical research techniques to CAM practices to investigate their safety and effectiveness. In the clinic, from both the doctors' and patients' points of view, keeping an open mind and communicating clearly about CAM is the best way to avoid danger from toxic or unproven CAM therapies.

Use of complementary and alternative medicine

Up to 50% of the Western population now use some form of CAM despite very few trials proving their beneficial effects. The single most commonly used CAM in most Western surveys is herbal medicine.

In patients with gastrointestinal complaints, CAM is most commonly used by those with irritable bowel syndrome and IBD.

Types of complementary and alternative therapy (derived from http://nccam.nih.gov. health.whatiscam)

Alternative medical systems

Complete systems of theory and practice:

* Homeopathy

* Naturopathy

list continues

---

* Traditional Chinese Medicine (including acupuncture)

* Ayurveda.

Mind–body interventions

Techniques to enhance the mind's capacity to affect bodily function:

* Hypnotherapy

* Creative therapies, e.g. art, music, dance.

Biologically based therapies

Use of naturally occurring substances:

* Herbal medicine.

Manipulative and body-based

Based on movement or manipulation of one or more parts of body:

* Chiropractic

* Osteopathy

* Reflexology

* Massage.

Homeopathy

The principle of homeopathy is to 'Treat like with like'. Tiny doses of potentially toxic materials, for example plant substances (e.g. belladonna, arnica), minerals (e.g. mercury, sulphur), or animal products (e.g. snake venom) are diluted to minute or even non-existent concentrations. They are then administered to a patient thought to be suffering with a symptom or disease that might be caused by that substance. The degree to which the dilution is taken means that not a single molecule of the original substance is likely to be present in the resulting medicine. Thus scientists have been sceptical of its possible effectiveness. There is no evidence that homeopathy works in IBD; however, some trials suggest that it may have benefits for other conditions (although many do not).

There are five NHS hospitals in UK that practise primarily homeopathic and other forms of complementary therapies. Homeopathy is also practised by a number of GPs.

Naturopathy

Naturopaths aim to improve health and treat disease by assisting the body's own ability to recover from illness and injury. It includes a broad array of CAM modalities, including manipulative and body-based therapies, herbalism, acupuncture, counselling, aromatherapy, nutrition, homeopathy, and so on.

Traditional Chinese Medicine and Qi

According to the ancient practice of Chinese Medicine, Qi is a vital energy force circulating the body between the major organs along meridians. There are 12 major meridians corresponding to the 12 major functions or organs of the body (which are not necessarily the same concept as bodily organs known in Western medicine). Qi must flow in the correct strength, direction, and quality through each meridian and organ for health to be maintained. Acupuncture points are located along the meridians and provide a means of altering the flow of Qi.

Illness occurs when there is a deficiency or excess of flow of Qi along the meridians.

Treatment is aimed at restoring healthy balance. This may take the form of traditional Chinese herbal medicine, acupuncture, or both.

Acupuncture

Acupuncture is becoming more widespread and is now also practised by Western doctors and practitioners. Although originally based in principles of traditional Chinese medicine, its effects, particularly on pain, are explainable by conventional science. In the West, it is used primarily for chronic pain syndromes, arthritis, allergies, and digestive disorders.

There is some evidence from trials that acupuncture works for pain relief, although not for giving up smoking. Problems with safety relate primarily to needle insertion causing injury and are likely to be minimized by careful practice. Sterile needles are, of course, imperative.

Moxibustion combines acupuncture with the burning of herbal concoctions at the blunt end of the needle.

Ayurveda

Ayurvedic medicine is an ancient system of healthcare that is native to the Indian subcontinent. 'Ayurveda' roughly translates as the 'knowledge of life'. It includes healthy living along with therapeutic measures that relate to physical, mental, social, and spiritual harmony. The most commonly practised Ayurvedic treatments in the West are massage, and dietary and herbal advice.

Hypnotherapy

Hypnosis is a natural state of heightened awareness, in which the mind is opened to beneficial suggestions. Therapeutic mental suggestions are introduced while you are in a relaxed and receptive state. Usually only light trances are induced and you remain aware of what's going on. The aim is to help to gain control over mental or physical processes. It is usually carried out one-to-one with a hypnotherapist. You may be given self-hypnosis exercises to use at home.

There is good evidence for safety and effectiveness of treatment of IBS with hypnotherapy. Studies in IBD are so far limited, but research is underway and preliminary results in the lab are encouraging.

Stages of hypnotherapy

Stage 1: Relaxation—gradual calming of the body and mind.

Stage 2: Deepening—counting down into an increasingly relaxed state.

Stage 3: Suggestion—repetition of positive statements related to intended goals, e.g. calming gut inflammation.

Stage 4: Ending—counting back into a fully alert state.

Herbal medicine

The use of plants for healing is an ancient tradition. Herbalists tend to use whole plant preparations rather than purified extracts. These may be used externally, on skin lesions or wounds, or internally as teas, tonics, or medicines. Many well known drugs used today were purified from plants, and drug companies maintain a keen interest in developing new agents from plants.

Osteopathy and chiropractic

These are manipulative therapies. Musculoskeletal misalignments or functional abnormalities are treated with manipulations of joints or muscles. The best known technique is the high velocity thrust to realign spinal or other joints. Initially these were used as complete systems of medicine but now practitioners tend to concentrate on musculoskeletal problems.

Reflexology

This is a manipulative/massage technique concerned with specific areas of the feet and hands corresponding to bodily organs.

Others

There are many other CAM techniques that are available. A good source of further information is http://www.nccam.nih.gov.health.whatiscam/.

Effective treatments for inflammatory bowel disease

Although limited, there are several published trials of CAM in IBD. These are listed in Table 10.1. These include Chinese herbal therapy with or without

Table 10.1 Trials of complementary and alternative therapy in active IBD showing some benefit

Ulcerative colitis treatments	Crohn's disease treatments
Jian Pi Ling tabs	Boswellia serrata
RSF-FS enemas	Acupuncture with moxibustion
Kui jie qing enemas	
Yukui tang tabs, herbal decoction enemas	
Aloe vera gel	
Wheat grass juice	
Germinated barley	
Boswellia serrata	
Acupuncture with moxibustion	
Bovine colostrums enemas	

RSF–FS: *Radix sophorae flavescentis* and *Flos sophorae*.

acupuncture, and other herbal therapies. It is important to note that the majority of these studies were performed in people with mild disease.

Advice if you are thinking about trying complementary and alternative medicine

Undoubtedly there are many unconventional approaches to treatment of IBD that work for individuals or even in many cases. However, it is worth remembering that so-called 'natural' therapies are not always safe and there are reports of significant poisoning effects of herbs and even lethal side-effects of some. Clearly, although all approaches are worth considering, safety must be the first priority.

Like all drugs, herbal medicines have the potential to be toxic and may interact with other drugs. Before taking them you are advised to discuss your case with your doctor and/or pharmacist. In addition, high velocity manipulative treatments may be ill-advised if you have osteoporosis.

As a general rule any claims for effective therapies are more reliable if they appear in independent publications, e.g. newspapers, NACC letters, etc. than if they are part of promotional literature for the product. It is also important never to stop your usual medication without consulting with your medical team first as this can sometimes be dangerous.

Of course, just because there is no published research on a CAM product or process does not mean that it does not work. It may only mean the trial has not been done.

Finding a complementary and alternative medicine practitioner

Most CAM practices are unregulated. However, registered practitioners are available in most modalities. We would recommend checking the registration of a practitioner before you use them.

The NHS in the UK provides some complementary therapies via a few GP surgeries and specialist 'Homeopathic' hospitals. You can ask your GP to consider a referral to such a hospital. These hospitals tend to provide a range of CAM rather than be restricted to homeopathy (which might be suggested by the name).

Conclusions

Up to 50% of patients with IBD have tried some form of CAM. Although there is a wide range of therapies available, there is a lack of reliable data about the efficacy and safety of most remedies. This is in part a consequence of the problems associated with designing and funding clinical trials involving CAM. As many patients with IBD use CAM it is important that research continues into its use. It is also important that CAM practices are regulated for their safety and quality.

Further education of doctors and other healthcare workers about the potential benefits and dangers of CAM is essential if they are to give well-informed advice to patients who are considering or already using CAM for their IBD.

11

Future and unproven treatments

> ## → Key points
>
> ◆ New drugs and treatments have to go through a rigorous testing process to prove that they work and are safe.
>
> ◆ Many drugs and treatments show early promise but only a few fulfil that promise when tested in randomized controlled trials.
>
> ◆ There is a vast amount of ongoing research into new treatments for inflammatory bowel disease.

Introduction

There is a constant stream of new treatments being developed for ulcerative colitis (UC) and Crohn's disease. These include new drugs, drugs that exist already for treatment of other conditions, new medical devices, and other novel ideas, like swallowing parasites!

The birth of new drugs

Before treatments become widely available and are accepted by the medical world, and before governments and health insurers will pay for them, they have to be proven effective and safe in properly designed and executed clinical trials. This is for several reasons.

In the early days of medicine, there was nothing to stop people selling *'Dr Quack's miracle cure-all'* (advertised with a few choice testimonials that could, of course, be entirely fabricated) to anyone who would buy it. You may think that this couldn't happen today, but there is a thriving industry of 'health providers' who will happily relieve sick and desperate people of their money with unproven and occasionally harmful therapies. To prevent this, in most countries, before drugs become available for prescription they have to be rigorously tested to prove that they work.

Second, trials must be performed to prove that treatments are safe, and to identify what side-effects can occur.

Third, treatments have to be proven cost-effective. This can be a trouble-some concept for both patients and doctors to accept on an individual basis. It is difficult to come to terms with the fact that a treatment that you know may work for you (or your patient) is deemed too expensive by a nameless bureaucrat. However, this is an important and inevitable part of healthcare provision today. Advances in medical science are so rapid that new ways of treating inflammatory bowel disease (IBD; and other conditions) are being developed all the time. Most of this comes from biotechnology and pharma-ceutical companies. Developing these treatments and putting them through tri-als is an extremely expensive process, particularly when you take into account the fact that only a fraction of new treatments make it through the rigorous testing process. The result of this is that when a new drug becomes available it is often very expensive (the company that developed it has to recoup its costs and make a profit—it is, after all, a company not a charity). This is not nor-mally a problem if the drug is effective for most people. Say a year's treatment with a new drug costs £10 000 (this is not unrealistic) *but* only works in 1 of 10 people treated. That means it costs £100 000 a year to help one person. If only 1 in 100 people respond, the cost is £1 million pounds per person helped. Of course, if you are that one person, then it is money well spent, but if you are a government or an insurance company, you wouldn't be so impressed. If all new treatments, however expensive and effective, were made freely available to all, governments and healthcare insurers would rapidly be bankrupted.

Why take part in a drug trial?

Many large hospitals run drug trials. These not only allow access to drugs that may not become available for many years, but also provide the department with extra funds that can be used for research or to employ, for example, an IBD nurse. But why do people with IBD take part in drug trials?

Perhaps most importantly, a drug trial may be the only way of getting access to a new and effective drug. For example, infliximab was given to hundreds of people in drug trials long before it was available to the general population. In addition, trials for new drugs are often designed to see if they can maintain IBD in remission. Therefore, the trials may last for up to a year. For people whose disease is poorly controlled, such trials potentially give access to a year of a new therapy. Even better, most drug companies understand that it would be unethical to withdraw a drug from a patient for whom it was working, just because the trial has finished. Therefore, many (but not all) trials have 'open label extensions'. In other words, if the drug works, the company will continue to give it to those people in the trial in whom it is effective, even after the trial has finished. This is important because drugs are often not approved for general use for months or years after trials have finished.

Of course, some people take part in drug trials simply to help. For example, drug trials may be designed to show that a new formulation of a well-established drug works. Obviously, drugs like these are unlikely to be vastly more effective than currently available treatments. They are usually developed to provide other benefits, such as taking the drug once as opposed to three times per day, or taking one as opposed to nine tablets a day. Drug companies are still obliged (quite rightly) to prove that the new formulation works—hence a trial. Unlike with new drugs, where the people recruited are likely to have active disease that hasn't responded to usual treatments, these trials may also recruit people whose disease is well controlled and stable.

What are the disadvantages of taking part in drug trials?

There is no guarantee that a trial drug will work. Having said this, before undergoing large-scale trials, drugs will have been through smaller trials that will have shown at least a suggestion that they are effective. They will also have been through rigorous safety testing, although this is no guarantee that people get no side-effects. The risks of trial drugs must also be considered in the light of the fact that all drugs used to treat IBD have some side-effects and many have potentially serious ones.

Taking part in drug trials also requires a certain amount of commitment on behalf of both the participant and their medical team. Trials normally mean appointments at least every few weeks (often more in the early stages of the trial and less later on). Participants will also be asked to fill out symptom diaries and have tests intermittently. These provide vital information about how effective the drug is and may also identify which patients are most likely to benefit from the drug.

Finally, in most trials of new drugs, there will be a placebo arm. That is, a randomly selected proportion of participants will receive a dummy drug, not the active version. This is the only way of proving that a drug works in diseases that can improve spontaneously, like Crohn's disease and UC. For an excellent description of placebo-controlled trials (written by a layman) see *Snake Oil and Other Preoccupations* by John Diamond (2001).

New treatments

It is inevitable that descriptions of upcoming treatments will quickly become out of date. Indeed, it may be of interest to those people reading this book in say 5 or 10 years time to consider how many (if any) of the following treatments have become accepted into mainstream practice. This may provide useful guidance into how to interpret the not infrequent articles found in some sections of the popular press proclaiming a miracle cure for IBD: rarely, if ever, do these stories come to much, and all too often they provide false hope. Far more reliable are reports found on the websites and in the newsletters of the patient support organizations (see Appendix 1) or those provided by reputable gastroenterological societies. Alternatively, if you feel so inclined, searching PubMed (http://www.pubmed.com) will provide abstracts of published research for you to interpret yourself.

Having said all of this, we have picked out some of the more interesting new treatments that are currently being investigated.

Parasites

Yes parasites! As discussed in Chapter 2, IBD is found more frequently in the Western world, but is now also becoming more common in the developing world. Infestation with parasites is found far more commonly in the developing world. However, as standards of hygiene increase and the rate of infestation falls, it has also become apparent that the prevalence of IBD is increasing. Thus, could it be that parasites may protect against the development of IBD?

This theory eventually led to trials using parasitic worms to treat people with IBD. The treatment involves drinking eggs (invisible to the naked eye) of a parasitic worm that normally infects pigs. The eggs then hatch in the small bowel, but in humans they are unable to infect the host. Instead they eventually pass out of the body in the faeces. However, their presence is enough to alter the way the immune system works and to improve the symptoms of IBD. In a relatively small placebo-controlled trial, the pork whipworm (*Trichuris suis*) was found to be slightly more effective than placebo in patients with UC. Although this is clearly not a miracle treatment for UC, it represents a fascinating advance in the treatment of IBD and it is possible that this pioneering work may go further. Of course, for some people, the idea of 'eating worms' is a step too far.

Leucocytapheresis

This technique originated in Japan where it is currently commonly used in the treatment of UC. Apheresis means 'taking away', and leucocytes are white blood cells. This treatment involves removing white blood cells from the blood, the cells responsible for inflammation. People receiving apheresis are attached to a machine that removes blood from a small needle in one arm, processes it, removing some of the white blood cells, and returns it to the other arm. The treatment lasts about an hour and is often given weekly in the first instance. Although apheresis is commonly used in Japan, it has yet to make a worldwide impact in the treatment of IBD as neither results of rigorous testing, nor the machinery to carry out the process are available. Results of bigger trials are, however, eagerly awaited—perhaps the leech-wielding doctors of yesteryear were on to something!

Appendectomy

Many years ago, researchers noted that people who had had their appendix removed were less likely to develop UC. This led to the theory that removal of the appendix (appendectomy) may help in patients with active UC. To date there is very little evidence to support this theory other than a small series of patients from Australia. Nevertheless, research into the role of the appendix in UC continues.

New drugs

There are far too many drugs being investigated as potential new treatments for IBD to list them all here. Instead we have picked out a few of the more interesting ones. These are at varying stages of investigation. Remember, history tells us that many drugs that show early promise fail to turn out to be as good as we hoped.

Areas of research in inflammatory bowel disease with some examples

♦ *New applications of old drugs*: naltrexone

♦ *New formulations of drugs used to treat IBD*: new release mechanisms for 5-aminosalicylic acids and steroids

♦ *New drugs*: new biologics

♦ *New therapeutic techniques*: apheresis

♦ *Complementary and alternative medicines*: hypnotherapy.

Naltrexone

This drug works on the same receptors that opioid painkillers (e.g. morphine) work on. A single study of 17 patients with Crohn's disease suggested that this drug was worth further investigation. It is currently undergoing further trials.

Viagra®

Amazing as it may sound, there are preliminary studies that show that, in theory, Viagra® (sildenafil) may be useful in the treatment of Crohn's disease. The researchers who discovered this are in the process of conducting a small clinical trial.

Antibiotics for *Mycobacterium avium paratuberculosis*

As discussed in Chapter 2, *Mycobacterium avium paratuberculosis* (MAP) has been, and remains, one of the great controversies in Crohn's disease. This has largely been fuelled by anecdotal reports of people responding to antibiotics that eradicate MAP. In 2007 a well conducted study from Australia suggested that anti-MAP treatment was not effective as a maintenance treatment for Crohn's disease, although enthusiasts for anti-MAP therapy have criticized the trial's design.

Cannabis

Preliminary results suggests that cannabinoids, one of the active components found in cannabis, may decrease inflammation in the bowel. Work in this area has led to a trial being conducted in Germany on the effects of cannabis in patients with Crohn's disease. To our knowledge, the results are, as yet, not available.

Conclusions

Over recent decades there have been a variety of exciting developments in the treatment of IBD. Both people with IBD and health professionals eagerly await further advances. However, due to the extensive testing needed to prove the efficacy and safety of new treatments, it is inevitable that their development is a slow process. It is also important to remember that for every new drug that makes it on to the market, thousands of people with IBD will have volunteered to take part in trials.

12

Diet and nutrition

> **→ Key points**
>
> ◆ With the exception of elemental and polymeric feeds for Crohn's disease, there is no specific dietary treatment that has been shown to improve inflammation in inflammatory bowel disease (IBD).
>
> ◆ Despite extensive research, diet has not been shown to play a direct role in causing IBD.
>
> ◆ Nevertheless, manipulation of the diet can improve symptoms in some people with IBD.
>
> ◆ Maintaining adequate nutrition and hydration is important in IBD.
>
> ◆ The role of probiotics and prebiotics in IBD is being investigated.

Questions about the role of diet and nutrition in inflammatory bowel disease (IBD) arise extremely commonly. This is unsurprising given that both are of immense importance in the management of IBD. Therefore, we have devoted an entire chapter to this subject.

Was it something I ate?

Before we address the subject of diet in greater detail, it is important to address this, perhaps the most commonly asked question, and to reiterate that diet is neither cause nor cure for IBD (see Chapter 2). Although many dietary components of diet have been proposed as a potential cause of IBD, none has been proven to cause either Crohn's or ulcerative colitis (UC). Given the enormous amount of research that has been conducted in this area, it seems unlikely that this will change. That is not to say, however, that diet cannot alter how active the disease is, or the sort of symptoms suffered.

Is there a diet that will reduce inflammation in inflammatory bowel disease?

For patients with Crohn's disease, particularly if it affects the small bowel, the short answer to this question is 'Yes'. In fact, in some parts of the world, nutritional therapy is used as a first-line treatment for children with Crohn's disease (see Chapter 8). The treatment involves taking drinks that contain all the basic components of a healthy diet (fat, protein, and carbohydrate) in their most simple forms. In other words, the diet consists of the basic building blocks of food from which our bodies manufacture all the compounds we need. Effectively, it is predigested food. These are known as elemental or polymeric diets and have been shown to decrease bowel inflammation in people with Crohn's disease. The downside to this form of treatment is that it seems to work best when all other food is excluded. This is perhaps one of the major reasons that it is rarely used in adults; in contrast to many children, adults are often unwilling to forfeit their favourite foods. Secondly, some (probably most) people do not like the taste of the drinks. One solution to this is to take the feed overnight through a nasogastric tube (a tube inserted through the nose into the stomach). Although inserting a tube through the nose into the stomach sounds fairly drastic, many children with Crohn's disease are able to master this simple technique themselves, allowing them to take out the tube each morning and put in a new one each night. Perhaps the biggest drawback, as with many treatments, is that the disease tends to recur when the treatment is stopped.

Experience of using this treatment in adults is limited, probably due to the problems outlined above. Nevertheless, some centres report that it works and is tolerable in adults as well as in children. Unfortunately, there is no dietary therapy that has been shown to reduce inflammation in patients with UC.

 Case study

Nutritional therapy

Jamie was 13 when he was diagnosed with Crohn's disease. He had been having crampy abdominal pains and diarrhoea for about a year before he was diagnosed. His specialist suggested to him that he try nutritional therapy. This was started while he was in hospital and, with the help of the nurses, he quickly learned how to pass the nasogastric tube himself. He carried on the treatment at home and was able to return to school. Although he sometimes missed normal food, he felt so much better on the nutritional therapy that he didn't mind, particularly as he started to grow and to catch up with his friends who had all been taller than him.

What about probiotics?

Probiotics are bacteria that are taken in an attempt to change the balance of the bacteria in the gut and thereby reduce inflammation (you will remember from Chapter 2 the important role played by the bacteria in the gut in IBD). Although it might seem strange to write about probiotics in a chapter covering diet and nutrition, many probiotics are sold in the form of yoghurt drinks, hence their inclusion here. In addition, there is developing interest in the role of *pre*biotics. These are substances taken in the diet that encourage the growth of specific bacteria in the gut that might improve inflammation. The fascinating and exciting area of prebiotics and probiotics is currently one of the most intensely researched subjects in IBD and has already produced some interesting results. For example, trials have shown that certain probiotics are as effective as 5-aminosalicylic acid drugs at preventing relapse in UC. Trials like these create much excitement and hope for the future. They are also useful, however, in helping us to understand where probiotics are likely to fit in with other treatments for IBD. At least for the moment, it appears that probiotics and prebiotics are likely to be treatments for mild or moderate IBD rather than for very severe disease.

Are there specific diets that can help to control my symptoms?

With some specific exceptions (see below) there are no hard and fast rules to follow here. In patients with UC, or with Crohn's disease of the colon, there should be no problem with absorption of food as the small bowel, which carries out this task, is unaffected. Therefore, as with anyone else, it is important to follow a balanced healthy diet. In general, the only dietary advice to follow is to avoid any foods that you find to worsen your symptoms. The easiest and simplest way to identify such foods is to keep a diet and symptom diary. However, this approach does not always work and eliminating foods from the diet is most safely and effectively done in conjunction with advice from a qualified dietician. This ensures that the diet is not too restrictive and contains sufficient energy along with all the necessary nutrients.

Dietary components that may exacerbate symptoms in inflammatory bowel disease

- Carbohydrates

  - small sugars—lactose, fructose, raffinose

  - larger carbohydrates—inulin, starch

  - sugar alcohols—sorbitol

- Alcohol

- Caffeine

- High fat foods

Many people find that diet has no effect on their symptoms. If it does, some of the substances listed above may be worth considering as potential factors.

Are there any particular culprits that are likely to cause me trouble?

Carbohydrates

In IBD, most symptoms are caused by inflammation, but some people find that reducing the amount of specific carbohydrates in the diet can help to decrease the amount of diarrhoea, wind, and bloating they get. Removing these foods from the diet, however, has no beneficial effect on the underlying inflammation.

Carbohydrates are an important part of our diet. Carbohydrate molecules vary in size from small (e.g. sugars such as sucrose, fructose, and lactose), through medium (e.g. raffinose) to large (e.g. inulin and starch). Digestion and absorption of carbohydrates varies from person to person. For example, while we can all absorb glucose easily, some of us are better at absorbing fructose than other people. Any carbohydrate that is not absorbed in the small bowel reaches the large bowel where it is fermented by bacteria.

Small sugars

Some people are unable to absorb lactose, the sugar present in milk. This is because they lack an enzyme called lactase that digests it. Lactase deficiency is much more common in certain racial groups (e.g. Asians) but is also probably slightly more common in people with Crohn's disease. People who are lactase deficient may benefit from only taking small amounts of lactose in the diet. Hard cheeses, live yoghurts, and cottage cheese contain only small amounts of lactose compared with milk and cream. It is also possible to buy milk with reduced quantities of lactose in it and soya milk is another alternative. Remember, however, that it is important to get enough calcium and vitamin D and that dairy products are one of the major sources of these substances in our diets.

Fructose is another sugar found in the diet. There is a limit to the amount of fructose we can absorb and, if we exceed that limit, some fructose will make it through to the large bowel potentially causing symptoms of bloating and wind. How much an individual can absorb varies from person to person and, probably also in the same person over time. For some people reducing the amount of fructose in the diet can help reduce some of the symptoms of IBD.

Larger carbohydrates

Large carbohydrates pass through our small bowel without being digested. This is because we lack the enzymes that break them down into smaller absorbable sugars. Foods such as cabbage, wheat, and onions are sources of these carbohydrates. When they reach the large bowel, they are rapidly fermented by the bacteria that live there and can worsen symptoms such as wind, bloating, and diarrhoea. This can happen in all people, whether they have IBD or not.

Caffeine and alcohol

Both caffeine and alcohol can worsen IBD symptoms in some people. Reducing intake of these substances, and only taking them in combination with food, may minimize these effects.

It is important to stress that dietary manipulation is not an alternative to treatment. With the exception of an elemental diet, changing what you eat does not affect the amount of inflammation in the bowel, it simply reduces dietary substances that can worsen symptoms. Second, as we shall discuss shortly, nutrition is of paramount importance in IBD and diets, which may be adequate for people without IBD, may not be right for you. A qualified dietician will be able to help make sure that you are getting all the nutrients you need as well as offering advice on symptom control.

How much fibre should I eat?

Fibre is an important component of our diet. Fibre is made up of various indigestible carbohydrates and is found in fruit, vegetables, pulses, nuts, and grains. It helps to keep stools soft and easy to pass. Some types of fibre add bulk to the stool while others are fermented by bacteria and encourage the growth of 'healthy' bacteria in the gut. It is also thought that some of the products of fermentation of fibre are important for a healthy colon. Therefore, for most people, whether they have IBD or not, it is important to have adequate intake of dietary fibre. There are, however, exceptions. The first is that fibre can worsen diarrhoea in people with active IBD. Some people find, therefore, that when their disease is active, it is easier for them to eat a low fibre diet. Second, fermentation of fibre leads to the production of gas. Therefore, people who get a lot of bloating sometimes find that their symptoms improve by decreasing the amount of fibre in their diet.

What about people with Crohn's disease of the small bowel?

Some people with Crohn's disease develop strictures (narrowings) in the small bowel. You will be aware of the fact that humans are unable to digest some foods. For example, sweetcorn passes through the body essentially unchanged—being bright yellow it can often be clearly seen in faeces. There are many such foods and, in people with strictures, they can become stuck. This leads to symptoms of crampy abdominal pain, nausea, and, if the blockage is severe, vomiting. Fortunately, these obstructions normally pass spontaneously, often with a loud rumbling/gushing sound from the abdomen. People who are known to have stricturing disease are often advised to eat a low fibre diet to avoid obstruction. Nuts, seeds, and some fruits and vegetables are examples of foods that should be avoided. Again, advice from a qualified dietician is the best way to get a good understanding of the diet while making sure that nutritional requirements are met.

People with small bowel Crohn's disease, particularly if it affects much of the bowel or if they have had some of the bowel removed, can sometimes have problems absorbing food. This can lead not only to inadequate nutrition and weight loss but can also worsen diarrhoea.

These people may find that foods high in fat are a particular problem and may complain of passing greasy foul-smelling stools. There are a variety of potential causes for this in Crohn's disease, some of which are reversible and some of which are not. Reducing the quantity of high fat and greasy foods in the diet is often the simplest way to improve symptoms.

Should I be taking supplements?

Most healthy people do not need to take supplements, so long as they are eating a balanced diet. However, it is undoubtedly true that people with IBD are at increased risk of becoming deficient in some vitamins and minerals.

Iron

Iron deficiency, for example, is common in people with IBD. Many multivitamin supplements bought in shops contain iron, although it is often in quantities that are too small to help. Therefore, iron tablets or liquid may need to be prescribed. Unfortunately, many people find that iron causes gastrointestinal side-effects when taken orally. There is also a proportion of people with IBD who find that oral iron supplements exacerbate their disease. Fortunately, infusions of iron are available that can be given easily and safely. These are so quick and effective that infusions are sometimes used in preference to oral iron supplements.

Vitamin B12

Another problem found in people with Crohn's disease is low levels of vitamin B12. This vitamin is found in foods such as meat, eggs, and dairy products. It is absorbed in the last part of the small bowel, the area most commonly affected by Crohn's disease. Therefore, in people with active inflammation in the terminal ileum, or in those who have had surgery to remove it, supplements of B12 may be required. These need to be given by injection, normally about four times a year.

Vitamin D

Vitamin D supplementation is also sometimes required. This is particularly important as people with IBD are at increased risk of thinning of the bones. In fact, many doctors will give supplements of calcium and vitamin D to protect the bones when people are taking steroids.

Folic acid

Folic acid is another vitamin that is frequently prescribed to people with IBD, particularly those taking drugs that interfere with its metabolism and/or absorption such as sulfasalazine and methotrexate. Of course, anyone thinking of becoming pregnant should be taking folic acid supplements whether they have IBD or not (see also Chapter 16).

Other vitamins and minerals

Except in patients with short bowel syndrome (see below) nutritional and vitamin deficiencies other than those described above are relatively uncommon.

Nutrition

The basic nutrients we require are fats, carbohydrates, and proteins. Each of these is an important part of our diet. As mentioned above, people whose Crohn's disease only affects their large bowel and people with UC should have no problem absorbing all the nutrients they need. Instead, dietary problems tend to arise due to under eating, either from lack of appetite or in an attempt to decrease the severity of diarrhoea. It is also important to remember that the body uses up slightly more energy when there is active inflammation in the bowel. This can mean that people with active IBD may be at even higher risk of undernutrition. Simple measures such as eating small amounts frequently and taking nutritional drinks may help in these circumstances.

When Crohn's disease affects the small bowel, or when some of the small bowel has been removed, problems with absorbing the required nutrients can arise. Although the term malnutrition often brings to mind television footage of famine victims, it is possible to be malnourished without such obvious changes in body shape. Symptoms of mild malnutrition can be subtle and non-specific and include tiredness, lack of energy, and increased susceptibility towards infection. Of course, the most obvious sign of malnutrition is weight loss. People at risk of malnutrition should be aware of weight loss. Weighing yourself occasionally and watching out for other signs, such as clothes or jewellery becoming loose fitting, are simple measures that can highlight the problem in its early stages.

Nutrition is of particular concern in children and adolescents with IBD as poor nutrition can lead to stunted growth and delayed puberty. This is a further reason why nutritional therapy is so popular in this age group: not only is it a treatment for Crohn's disease but it also improves the nutritional state.

Short bowel syndrome

Rarely, there is not enough functioning small bowel to absorb all the nutrients needed. This is most commonly seen in patients with Crohn's disease who have had a series of operations and have eventually had much of their small bowel removed. This condition is called intestinal failure or short bowel syndrome and, fortunately, is very rare. People with short bowel syndrome may rely on intravenous feeding (directly into a vein) to get their required nutrients. Technology in this field has advanced to such an extent over recent decades that there are now hundreds of people in the UK who live in their own homes and lead normal lives surviving entirely on intravenous feeding.

Keeping well hydrated

Maintaining hydration is also an important consideration for people with IBD, particularly if they have diarrhoea. Dehydration causes non-specific symptoms including tiredness and weakness. Hot weather can exacerbate the problem. Drinking rehydration solutions that contain salt and glucose is the safest way to rehydrate, although for most people, simply being aware of the risk of dehydration and drinking regularly is sufficient. People with short bowel syndrome need to be aware that drinking water without added salt and sugar can worsen dehydration; your healthcare team will tell you if this applies to you. People who have had a colectomy are also prone to dehydration as they can lose a lot of salt and water through the stoma or pouch.

Conclusions

Knowing what and how much to eat can be one of the greatest challenges for people with IBD. The best people to advise on diet are qualified dieticians, particularly those who have an interest in IBD. Excluding foods on a trial and error basis and the use of food diaries can also provide useful information. Finally, listening to the experience of other people with IBD may also be helpful.

13

Complications and extraintestinal manifestations

⊋ Key points

◆ About a quarter of people with inflammatory bowel disease get an extraintestinal manifestation.

◆ These commonly affect the bones and joints, the skin and the eyes.

◆ Less commonly, other organs may be affected.

◆ People frequently get more than one extraintestinal manifestation.

Inflammatory bowel disease (IBD) can cause problems outside the guts. These are called extraintestinal manifestations (EIMs). Some are common and others are very rare. Sometimes they are a complication of IBD, resulting from the disease itself, for example, anaemia and osteoporosis. In other cases, there seems to be a genetic or pathological association with IBD.

About 1 in 4 people with IBD develop EIMs. It also appears that if you have one EIM you are at higher risk of getting another. For some reason, people whose IBD predominantly affects the colon also seem to be at higher risk of getting EIMs.

Joint and bone disease

Enteropathic arthropathy

This describes a form of arthritis that is found specifically in people with IBD. It affects about 10% of people with IBD and may take several forms.

Table 13.1 Common extraintestinal manifestations and complications of IBD

Joints and bones	Enteropathic arthropathy
	Sacroilietis
	Ankylosing spondylitis
	Osteoporosis
Skin	Erythema nodosum
	Pyoderma gangrenosum
Eyes	Episcleritis
	Uveitis
Liver and biliary tract	Cholesterol gallstones
	Primary sclerosing cholangitis
Blood	Anaemia
	Venous and arterial thrombosis
Mouth	Aphthous ulceration
	Orofacial granulomatosis
Constitutional	Weight loss
	Growth retardation
Malignancy	Bowel cancer
	Lymphoma
Kidneys	Oxalate stones
	Uric acid stones

Peripheral arthritis

Type 1

One or a few large joints are affected. For example, people with this form of arthritis may develop a hot swollen ankle or knee. Attacks tend to coincide with a relapse of IBD and may be associated with other EIMs such as erythema nodosum or iritis (see below).

Type 2

Multiple small joints are affected. For example, people with this form of arthritis may develop inflammation of the joints in the fingers. This can be a more chronic problem, not necessarily related to activity of the underlying IBD and usually needs treatment in addition to that being used for IBD.

Axial disease

Ankylosing spondylitis affects about 5% of patients with IBD. It presents with back pain and stiffness, often in the lower back. Activity is not related to the bowel inflammation. Treatment is with physiotherapy, anti-inflammatories, or sometimes infliximab. Sacroilietis is another form of axial arthritis that only affects the sacroiliac joints.

Which drugs are used to treat arthritis in IBD depends on whether activity of the arthritis follows that of the underlying IBD. If it does, then treating the bowel inflammation is normally enough. In many people, changing their 5-amino salicylic acid drug to sulfasalazine (which was originally developed as a drug for people with arthritis—see Chapter 8) is often helpful. Steroids may also be used to treat arthritis.

Non-steroidal anti-inflammatories, such as ibuprofen, are excellent painkillers for people with arthritis. Unfortunately, these drugs can make IBD worse in some people. Therefore, if possible, they are avoided in IBD.

Osteoporosis

Osteoporosis is a generalized thinning of the bones, which leads to an increased risk of fracture. Bones thin gradually with age and lack of exercise, which is why older people are more likely to get fractures if they fall over. In IBD this thinning can occur more rapidly as a consequence of the intestinal inflammation, inability to absorb nutrients, and treatment with steroids. The risk of getting osteoporosis increases the more steroids are used and becomes much more likely once about seven to eight courses have been given. Many doctors will prescribe calcium and vitamin D tablets with every course of steroids to try to prevent osteoporosis.

Osteoporosis does not cause any symptoms unless a fracture occurs and there is no way of knowing that you are developing it without regular scans. Therefore, people at high risk of developing osteoporosis should have bone densitometry (DEXA) scanning every few years to check for osteopenia (an early sign of osteoporosis) or for osteoporosis. This can be treated with calcium and vitamin D supplements, and sometimes needs more specific treatment. If you have never had a bone density scan it is worth mentioning at your next appointment to remind your doctor you might need one.

Smoking also worsens osteoporosis. This is yet another reason to give up!

Skin

Erythema nodosum is a condition that occurs when IBD is active. About 8% (1 in 12) of people with IBD get erythema nodosum at some point. Hot, red-purplish tender nodules about 1–2 cm in size, appear on the shins although rarely they can occur elsewhere. Sometimes, erythema nodosum is associated with a swollen and painful joint or two. Treatment of the active IBD is often all that is needed. The swellings last a few days and gradually fade.

Pyoderma gangrenosum is an ulcerating skin condition that occurs in 2% (1 in 50) of people during the course of their IBD. It is not related to active bowel inflammation. Initially a single pustule (white headed spot) with a surrounding red area develops anywhere on the body, most commonly the legs. The top then blackens, ulcerates, and enlarges. Without treatment, it doesn't heal. Sometimes pyoderma gangrenosum can become very large and very painful without treatment. Rarely there can be several lesions. The most effective treatment is infliximab, although a variety of ointments are sometimes tried first.

Eyes

Episcleritis and uveitis are inflammatory conditions affecting the eyes. People with episcleritis or uveitis will complain of red sore eyes. Anyone who develops these symptoms should see an eye specialist to have a full examination as very rarely these conditions can affect eyesight if left untreated.

Liver and biliary tract

Primary sclerosing cholangitis

This condition affects the biliary tree. The biliary tree is a system of canals and ducts that drains bile produced by the liver and takes it to the intestine where it helps to digest fat. It starts with small branches that join together to form larger branches and, eventually, a single main trunk. Hence the term 'tree'.

Primary sclerosing cholangitis (PSC) occurs in up to 5% (1 in 20) of people with ulcerative colitis although it is less common in people with Crohn's disease. It can occur even before colitis develops. There is gradual progressive narrowing of the ducts causing blockage to bile flow. In the early stages, the only abnormality is in liver blood tests. Later, jaundice and cirrhosis can develop.

People with IBD who develop abnormal liver blood tests may require further investigations with, for example, liver ultrasound and/or an MRI scan. This is the easiest and safest way of detecting early signs of PSC. Treatment is with ursodeoxycholic acid tablets to try to prevent progression, but careful monitoring is still needed. Some patients may eventually require a liver transplant. There are patient support groups for people with PSC (see Appendix 1).

PSC is also associated with an increased risk of bowel cancer and, therefore, anyone with PSC will be offered a yearly colonoscopy to check for early signs of cancer (see below).

Gallstones

Gallstones are stones that form in the gallbladder. The gall bladder is a bag that is connected to the biliary tree (see Fig. 13.1). It stores bile until we eat something, when it contracts ejecting its contents into the intestine to help digest fat. Gallstones are very common, but people with Crohn's disease, are at increased risk of developing gallstones. This is particularly true if the terminal ileum is diseased or has been removed, Most gallstones do not cause symptoms and do not need treatment. However, they can cause a variety of problems, including pain and jaundice. In such cases, they are best treated by surgery.

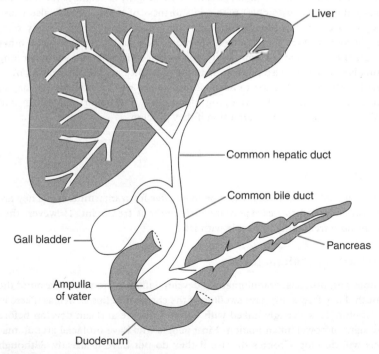

Figure 13.1 Biliary tree and gall bladder.

Blood

Anaemia

Anaemia can occur for a variety of reasons in IBD. Blood loss from the bowel wall is the most common cause. Sometimes this can occur without the blood being visible in the stool. Poor absorption of vitamins (for example, B12 and folate) and/or of iron can also contribute to anaemia. Although mild anaemia may not cause symptoms, as it becomes more severe, it can cause shortness of breath and tiredness (see Chapter 4). Anaemia should be treated, as treatment can improve symptoms and quality of life markedly.

Venous and arterial thrombosis

Deep vein thrombosis (DVT) and pulmonary embolism are the best known examples of these conditions. In DVT, a clot forms in one of the large veins, most commonly in the legs. This causes redness and painful swelling of the affected leg. Pulmonary embolism occurs when a bit of clot breaks away from a DVT and travels in the blood stream to the lungs. This condition can be life threatening and causes chest pain and shortness of breath. It may also cause people to cough up blood. Although these conditions are relatively rare, people with IBD are about three times more likely to develop them than other people. Long periods of immobility, for instance after operations or on long haul plane journeys, also predispose to these conditions. For this reason, most people with IBD admitted to hospital receive heparin injections every day to decrease the chance of developing blood clots. Pulmonary embolism and DVT need urgent medical attention if they develop.

Mouth

Aphthous ulceration

These are small ulcers that most people suffer from intermittently. They are painful and tend to heal spontaneously without treatment. However, they occur more frequently in people with IBD.

Orofacial granulomatosis

People with orofacial granulomatosis develop inflammation in and around the mouth. They frequently have swelling of the cheeks and lips as well as ulcers in the mouth. It is strongly linked with Crohn's disease and can develop before any signs of bowel inflammation. Most people who have orofacial granulomatosis will develop Crohn's disease if they do not have it already. Although medication may be effective, dietary restriction of foods containing cinnamon or benzoate (an additive often found in soft drinks) may also improve the condition.

Malignancy

Bowel cancer

There is an increased risk of bowel cancer in patients with IBD if it affects most of the colon (i.e. extensive ulcerative colitis and Crohn's colitis). The risk of developing bowel cancer increases gradually with time. However, the risk is still small. Cancer can start with a small patch of abnormal cells (dysplasia) in the colon. To try to reduce the risk of people with IBD developing cancer, regular colonoscopies are performed in those who are at high risk of developing it (i.e. people with extensive colonic disease for more than 10 years). This is known as surveillance colonoscopy. Lots of biopsies are taken during a very careful examination of the colon to look for areas of dysplasia and sometimes dye is sprayed on to the bowel wall to highlight abnormalities. The interval between colonoscopies varies but is normally between a year and 5 years. People with PSC are at particularly high risk and most have yearly examinations as soon as their PSC is diagnosed. If dysplasia is detected in the biopsy samples you will probably be advised to have an operation to remove the entire colon. This prevents cancer developing and can, therefore, be life-saving.

Lymphoma

It is still unclear whether there is an increased risk of lymphoma in people with IBD. As we discussed in Chapter 8, the issue is confused by the fact that certain drugs, such as azathioprine are also associated with an increased risk of developing lymphoma. If IBD *is* associated with lymphoma, the remaining uncertainty about the link tells us one thing—the increased risk of developing this relatively rare form of cancer must be small.

Kidneys

IBD is associated with an increased risk of developing kidney stones. The reasons behind this are complicated but relate in part to changes in absorption of various minerals. This, combined with dehydration and an alteration in the acidity of the urine, both of which can occur in people with IBD, predisposes to the development of kidney stones. Kidney stones predispose people to developing urinary tract infections. If a stone becomes stuck in the tubes connecting the kidneys to the bladder it causes a severe pain known as renal colic. Occasionally, kidney stones may be associated with blood in the urine.

Constitutional

Weight loss

This is a common finding in people with active IBD and is due to a combination of some or all of the following: poor appetite, malabsorption, and active inflammation. The importance of nutrition is discussed in Chapter 12.

Growth retardation

The reasons for growth retardation in children with IBD are similar to those described in the previous paragraph. However, delayed puberty and use of steroids can be added as potential causes of growth retardation. This is discussed further in Chapter 15.

Conclusions

There is a wide variety of conditions associated with IBD, some of which flare up with the underlying disease and some of which don't. We have discussed most of the commoner EIMs, although there are several rarer conditions that we have not mentioned.

14

What can I do to help myself?

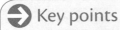 Key points

* Helping yourself can help you to feel in control of your disease.

* Patient support groups, such as the NACC, CCFA, and ACCA provide information and support from a patient's perspective.

* Stopping smoking is very important if you have Crohn's disease.

Introduction

Part of learning to live with a chronic illness involves not allowing it to control your life. This does not mean going into denial and pretending that you don't have inflammatory bowel disease (IBD), but rather continuing to live a normal life *with* IBD. An important component of this for many people is to do all they can to help themselves. In this chapter, we look at some of the things that you might want to do that fit into the category of 'helping yourself'. Of course, not all things suit all people and some of the following are more important than others. Nevertheless, we hope it might at least provide some food for thought.

Join a patient association

The development of patient associations, such as the NACC (UK), CCFA (USA), and ACCA (Australia) (see Appendix 1) has had positive effects both directly and indirectly for people with IBD. These organizations are a valuable source of information and support. Because they are run with and by people with IBD, not by healthcare professionals, they are focused on patient support from a patient's point of view. For example, every member of the NACC, the UK patient association for people with IBD, receives

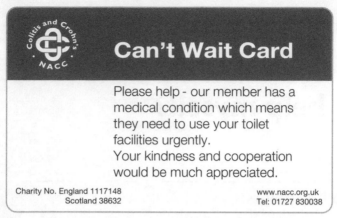

Figure 14.1 'Can't Wait Card' as provided on the back of the NACC membership card.

a 'Can't Wait Card' (Fig. 14.1), the potential benefit of which is self-explanatory.

Patient associations are valuable sources of information about all sorts of challenges that people with IBD may face. For example, they can suggest companies to approach for travel insurance. They are also able to offer information about welfare benefits that may be available to people with IBD and how to claim for them.

Although not run by doctors, these organizations tend to work closely with healthcare professionals who treat people with IBD. This ensures that accurate medical information is provided, for example, about medication and surgery.

The role of patient associations goes far beyond these examples. They also raise money to support research (both authors have been lucky enough to receive research grants from NACC). They can also be powerful and highly effective lobbying organizations. For example, the NACC recently ran a campaign to increase awareness of the importance of IBD nurses, putting pressure on local and national health agencies to provide funding. This has very real potential benefits for people with IBD. Finally, through local groups, patient associations often create strong social networks, which, as well as being good fun, can also be very supportive at times of need.

By definition, patient associations rely on the dedication and hard work of their members. So if you haven't joined your local or national association, please consider it (names and contact details can be found in Appendix 1).

Patient's perspective

Some comments from an NACC member:

The NACC provides clear and easy to understand information on IBD and its treatment.

I always look forward to receiving my newsletter, which details current research projects and fundraising events, gives tips and advice from other patients, and has a question and answer section. I enjoy reading every page and find it makes me feel less isolated.

I attend my local Support Group and find it beneficial to talk to other people who have IBD.

In addition to providing information, the NACC website has a discussion forum for young people. It is a great place to ask questions, post experiences, and generally be one of the community.

If you have Crohn's disease, stop smoking

In Chapter 2, we discussed the harmful effects of smoking in people with Crohn's disease. We also discussed the beneficial effects of giving up smoking. To remind you, these include an improvement in disease activity and symptoms, an improvement in the effectiveness of some drugs and a decreased chance of needing surgery. If you are a smoker who has Crohn's disease, this is the most important and effective thing that you can do that will alter your disease.

Of course, additional benefits of giving up smoking, include a decreased risk of developing heart disease, chronic lung disease, and a variety of cancers, not just lung cancer. For these reasons, people with ulcerative colitis should also consider giving up smoking. There are also obvious financial benefits.

Needless to say most people do not find giving up smoking easy. Having a good reason to stop is important, and having Crohn's disease is a *very* good reason to give up smoking. Many hospitals now have smoking cessation clinics and it may be possible for you to be referred to one of these. Some people find nicotine replacement helpful, for example as gum or patches, while others have success simply going 'cold turkey'. There are plenty of self-help guides to giving up smoking and some people swear by these. Whatever your chosen method, it's never too late to try. If you've failed before, don't let that prevent you from trying again—next time it may work.

Finally, if you needed any further persuasion, there is now some suggestion that passive smoking in childhood may predispose to the development of IBD. Sometimes it's easier to do something for someone else than for yourself!

Take your medication

We all know that taking medication every day can be both difficult and tedious. This is often particularly so for those drugs that are used to prevent relapse but seem to have no immediate benefit. Other drugs may take weeks or months to work, while some may have either annoying or unpleasant side-effects. Understanding what your medication is for and how it works, along with ways to minimize side-effects may make taking it easier. In addition, making your medication part of your daily life, for example taking it at mealtimes, or as part of your getting up or going to bed routine may also help you remember to take your drugs. Some people use dosette boxes, in which tablets are kept in separate compartments labelled with the day and time they are to be taken. If you are having trouble taking your medication, for whatever reason, talk to your medical team or pharmacist.

Of course, not all drugs are right for everyone and it can often take several changes of medication before you find the right combination. Perhaps most important of all, if you decide you want to discontinue one or all of your drugs, it is important that you discuss it with a member of your healthcare team. In some cases, it may actually be dangerous for you to stop a drug suddenly (see Chapter 8). It is, therefore, important that you feel able to talk openly with your doctors and nurses. For this to happen, you need to do the following.

Build a good relationship with your healthcare team

We hope that most healthcare professionals are sympathetic and easy to get on with. Nevertheless, there are bound to be some people that you find it easier to talk to than others. For example, you may find it easier to talk about personal things with someone of the same sex. Most healthcare teams looking after people with IBD are made up of both men and women and are sensitive to these issues. Remember too that primary care doctors (GPs) are an important part of the team. Some people have known their 'family doctor' for many years and are happier discussing certain issues with them rather than with their specialist.

Easy access to medical advice is vital for people with IBD. Many hospitals have helplines that you can use to contact your team in-between appointments (see Chapter 7). A judiciously timed phone call may prevent an unnecessary trip to the clinic or even a flare-up. Most importantly, if there are things you feel you need to discuss with a healthcare professional, make sure you do so sooner rather than later.

Plan ahead

Although there is no reason why people with IBD cannot lead a normal life, at times, life is easier with a little planning ahead. Knowing the location of public facilities or having a few trusted friends or relatives who do not mind you popping in to use their toilet can be very helpful if you are going out, particularly during a flare.

Similarly, thinking ahead about holidays; making sure you have adequate supplies of medication, knowing what you will do if you have a flare-up while away and thinking about travel insurance well in advance are all worthwhile. The last thing you want is to be worried and stressed about these things the day before you leave on your well earned break.

Some people carry a change of clothes with them if their disease is particularly active; although they may well not need to use them, the security of having them available can give people the confidence to do things they may otherwise avoid.

Be positive

The importance of having a positive approach cannot be underestimated. This is easier said than done at times. However, trying to think about things in a positive manner will not only be good for you mentally, but may well also help you feel better physically. Being positive includes recognizing your successes, not only in relation to your disease but also in life itself. Enjoying yourself and not allowing your life to be controlled by your illness will help you to feel positive. Humour is also a very useful tool for dealing with adversity. Sometimes having a good laugh about a difficult or embarrassing situation is the best way to cope with it!

Don't expect too much from yourself

Conversely, you should not expect too much of yourself. When your disease is active, make sure you allow yourself enough time for rest and recuperation. Similarly, allow yourself time to recover from flares or surgery – it can take weeks or even months to recover fully from an operation or a bad flare-up. Recognize too that at times you may feel depressed and angry. You may wonder why you were the one who was unlucky enough to get IBD. These are normal reactions and you should not feel guilty about having them. We are all human and have our bad days as well as our good.

Avoid stress

In Chapter 2 we discussed the role that stress may play for some people with IBD. If you find that stress exacerbates your disease then you should try to reduce the amount of stress in your life. Although it is impossible to lead a stress-free life, there are various things that you can do to help (see box below). It is also important to make the most of your free time. Taking holidays, spending quality time with family and friends, and sometimes just doing nothing are all important ways of helping us deal with the stresses of life. Relaxation techniques and meditation, although not for everyone, may also be helpful.

Dealing with stress: tips for work and home

◆ Try to identify what causes you stress.

◆ Plan ahead for events that you know will be stressful—being prepared for them may help minimize the stress they cause.

◆ Don't take on too much and know your limits. Be prepared to say 'No'.

◆ Try to manage your time effectively.

◆ Delegate—if you don't have to do something, ask someone else to do it.

Eat sensibly

We devoted an entire chapter to the importance of diet and nutrition in IBD (Chapter 12). Avoiding foods that exacerbate your symptoms while ensuring you eat enough to keep you healthy gives you the best chance of coping with a flare-up. It is also important to avoid dehydration, something that people with active IBD are particularly prone to. Finally, when travelling abroad, if water hygiene cannot be relied on, take sensible precautions such as peeling fruit, drinking bottled water, and avoiding salads (which will most likely have been washed in tap water) to minimize the risk of food poisoning. This would not only spoil your holiday but might initiate a relapse of your IBD.

Take exercise

Keeping active is not only good for us physically, but also mentally. Of course, active IBD can affect people's ability to exercise and sometimes it is simply impossible to get the energy up to do things. Also, exercise can make people need to open their bowels.

However, particularly for those in remission or with mild disease, getting out of the house and into natural light and fresh air often makes people feel better. There has even been some recently published research showing that light exercise improves the quality of life of people with mild or inactive Crohn's disease. Importantly, exercise may also help to decrease the risk of developing osteoporosis.

Minimizing the risk of osteoporosis

In Chapter 13 we discussed the fact that people with IBD are at increased risk of developing osteoporosis. Here are several simple steps that decrease this risk.

◆ Stop smoking

◆ Take weight-bearing exercise

◆ Do not drink excessive amounts of alcohol

◆ Make sure you are getting enough calcium (1–1.5 g per day) and vitamin D in your diet. Foods rich in calcium include, milk and dairy products, salmon and sardines, white and baked beans, and many green vegetables. Exposure to sunlight is our main source of vitamin D. It is also possible to get some in our diet by eating foods such as fatty fish, liver, and egg yolks. Also, some foods are now fortified with calcium and vitamin D and, if needed, supplements are available.

Find someone you can confide in

Perhaps most important of all you should try to find someone that you can talk to. This may be your partner, a family member, or a close friend. Often simply talking about a problem or how you are feeling is enough to make things seem better. Simple sensitive advice or reassurance can put seemingly insurmountable problems into perspective. A friendly, trusting, confidential ear may be all that is needed to make your concerns simply fade away. One thing is for sure, talking about a problem is unlikely to make it worse.

Conclusions

Taking control of your illness, rather than allowing it to control you, helps people to live with their IBD. Helping yourself is an important part of this, as is allowing others to help you.

15

Inflammatory bowel disease in childhood and adolescence

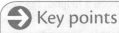 Key points

- Inflammatory bowel disease (IBD) is frequently diagnosed in childhood and adolescence.

- Although IBD is essentially the same disease whether it affects children or adults, there may be additional challenges faced by children with IBD and by their families.

- IBD can have both physical and psychological effects on young people.

- Children and adolescents with IBD may also face social challenges.

Introduction

Inflammatory bowel disease (IBD) typically first presents in childhood or early adult life. Although it can occur in very young children it is rare for it to be diagnosed before the age of 2. The management of IBD is very similar in children and adults; however, some of the challenges faced by young people with IBD, and by their families and medical teams are slightly different.

One of the biggest fears of young people with IBD is whether they can lead a normal life. Fortunately, all but a tiny minority of people are able to control their disease and remain symptom-free for most of the time.

Specialists who look after children with IBD are aware of the special challenges faced by people who grow up with Crohn's or ulcerative colitis (UC). One of these relates to the transition from paediatric to adult medical services that occurs in the late teens. It can be difficult to leave behind the healthcare team that has looked after you, sometimes for many years, and to build a relationship with a new team. In some centres there are crossover clinics attended by both the paediatric and adult teams to help people through this transition period.

School and education

Many children and adolescents with IBD (and their families) worry about the effect that the disease will have on their education. Sometimes, particularly during a flare, people do not feel well enough to attend school. Also, the symptoms of active IBD, such as abdominal pain, fatigue, and anaemia can affect concentration. Exam times are often particularly worrying.

There are various strategies to deal with these issues. Staying in touch with the school during periods of extended absence or hospitalization is helpful. Teachers may be able to send work home or get classmates to deliver it. The latter has the advantage of maintaining social contact with school friends. Sometimes extra tuition may help people to catch up on missed work. Examination Boards may allow extra time and different examination conditions for people with IBD. You will probably need a letter from your gastroenterologist to the school and/or examination board to get special dispensation for this.

Going to school can also create other challenges. Frequent trips to the toilet, embarrassment about using shared toilets and fear of having accidents may all concern young people with IBD. Understandably, some people worry about having to explain their condition to their classmates and teachers. Bullying (and the fear of it) can be particularly difficult to deal with. Sensitive action by schools with regard, for example, to toilet facilities and a place to store a change of clothes can help. Education of pupils and staff about the disease may be useful, although this has to be weighed against an individual's wish not to tell everyone about their condition and their right to privacy. It can be difficult to know who to tell and who not to. At school, it is probably wise to have at least one teacher who is aware of the diagnosis and to whom a child can talk openly about how they are feeling.

Fortunately, the general public's knowledge about IBD and the difficulties faced by young people with Crohn's and UC, has increased rapidly over the last few years, particularly within the education system. In particular this is due to the admirable efforts of the patient associations, such as the NACC and CCFA, who have raised overall awareness about IBD. They have produced a variety of helpful booklets and advice sheets. For example, both the NACC and CCFA produce excellent information leaflets (available from their websites) directed at schools and teachers.

Remember, IBD is a common condition and many schools will have at least one pupil who has either Crohn's or UC.

Symptoms and signs of inflammatory bowel disease in children

IBD, in particular Crohn's disease, can be difficult to diagnose in children. This is because most children get abdominal symptoms such as diarrhoea and abdominal pain from time to time. It is, therefore, easy to dismiss these symptoms or put them down to childhood infections. For example, Crohn's disease in children is not infrequently diagnosed at operations that are being done because of a presumed diagnosis of appendicitis. To make matters more difficult, it is not uncommon for children with Crohn's disease to present without a history of diarrhoea, one of the typical symptoms of IBD. By contrast, children with UC nearly always develop bloody diarrhoea.

Different presenting symptoms and signs of IBD in children are listed in the box below.

Symptoms and signs of inflammatory bowel disease in children

- Growth delay

- Weight loss

- Delayed puberty

- Abdominal pain

- Abdominal mass

- Diarrhoea

- Rectal bleeding

- Perianal abscesses and/or fistulae

- Oral symptoms—ulceration/facial or lip swelling

- Joint inflammation

- Fever

Oral Crohn's disease

Crohn's disease affecting the mouth is uncommon, although it is not unusual for people to get oral manifestations of Crohn's disease such as aphthous ulcers. True oral Crohn's disease, like Crohn's disease elsewhere in the gastrointestinal tract, is diagnosed by taking biopsies. It normally causes swelling of the lips and/or cheeks. These changes can, in fact, occur without any other signs of inflammation in the gut. When this occurs, the condition is known as OFG (orofacial granulomatosis). Oral Crohn's disease and OFG are much more common in young people than in adults. Many of the usual IBD treatments are used to treat oral Crohn's disease. However, this is another condition that to responds to dietary manipulation. Cutting out foods containing cinnamon aldehyde (a flavouring) and benzoates (a preservative) can be the most effective treatment.

Investigation of inflammatory bowel disease in children and adolescents

Tests used to investigate children with IBD are very similar to those used in adults (see Chapter 5). Although most adolescents can tolerate endoscopic procedures with sedation, younger children normally have these performed under general anaesthetic. Many children (and adults!) find the medication taken the day before the colonoscopy to ensure the bowel is empty, often called 'bowel prep', worse than the procedure itself.

Some children find that the amount of fluid they are required to swallow for tests such as a barium follow through, is too much for them. If this is a problem, a small tube passed through the nose into the stomach or small bowel may help. As discussed in Chapter 5, the role of capsule endoscopy in IBD is evolving. This may become a more commonly used test in the future.

Treatment of inflammatory bowel disease in children and adolescents

Chapter 8 describes medications used in the management of IBD. Most of the drugs prescribed for adults may also be used in children. Needless to say, the doses may differ. Perhaps the biggest difference in management strategies between children and adults is the use of nutritional therapy for people with Crohn's disease. This is used far more commonly in children than in adults for reasons discussed in Chapters 8 and 12.

Of particular concern to many children and their families is the safety of the drugs used to treat IBD. Although all drugs have potential side-effects, as long as medication is taken in the prescribed manner and monitored correctly, it is generally safe. It is important to understand the risks and benefits of all treatments compared with the alternatives, such as surgery or no treatment at all. An example of this is the use of steroids in children. Steroids are known to cause slowing of growth. However, as active disease also causes growth failure, treatment with steroids can actually increase growth rather than delay it by inducing remission of the disease. In these circumstances, the risks of growth retardation caused by the steroids are outweighed by the benefits on growth of getting the disease controlled. This is just one example of weighing up the pros and cons of treatment. Spending some time talking about these things with your specialist before starting new treatments is time well spent.

Surgery in children

Most children with IBD do not require operations but, in a small proportion, surgery is the best option. In children with UC, this will involve colectomy (removal of the colon—see Chapter 9). This operation is also sometimes performed on people with Crohn's disease affecting the large bowel. After the operation the person is left with a stoma. In some people it is possible to rejoin the bowel at a later date. Before surgery, both the child and their family should have the opportunity to discuss the operation with a surgeon and with a nurse who specializes in looking after people with stomas, often called a Stoma Therapist. Most children cope with having a stoma without any problem and the vast majority feel much better after their diseased bowel has been removed. In addition, most will be able to stop some or all of their treatment.

In children with a short segment of small bowel affected by Crohn's disease, surgery is sometimes preferred to drug treatment as it induces remission very quickly. This returns the child to good health and a normal life rapidly, whereas persisting with drug therapy may delay this. Sometimes surgery is the fastest way to catch up on delayed growth and development (see Fig. 15.1).

Surgery for Crohn's disease may also be indicated if there is a stricture in the bowel or there is active disease that fails to respond to treatment. Timing of surgery can often be organized to suit school and exam commitments. For example, a child with a flare of Crohn's could be treated with nutritional therapy to improve their symptoms and nutrition while sitting their exams. They could then have an operation during the summer holidays, leaving them fit for the next term without missing any school at all.

135

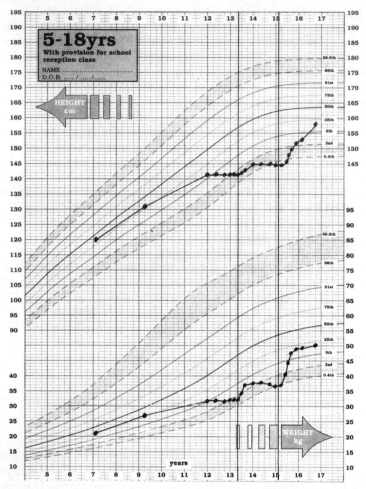

Figure 15.1 The growth chart of a girl with Crohn's disease. Note how the weight (bottom line) and height (top line) stop increasing at about age 12. The diagnosis was made at 13 (first vertical line) when nutritonal therapy was started. This was followed by an improvement in symptoms with some catch-up growth. However, as can be seen the disease relapsed. The second vertical line indicates surgery (right hemicolectomy) and is followed by remission and catch-up growth.

Eating and growth

In Chapter 12, we discussed the importance of diet and nutrition in people with IBD. Making sure that children with IBD get enough nutrition is possibly even more important than it is in adults. This is because inadequate nutrition can delay growth and development. That is why doctors who specialize in looking after young people with IBD will record their height and weight periodically on a growth chart (see Fig. 15.1). They will also take careful note of the child's development and progression through puberty. It is crucial that children get enough nourishment to allow them to grow. Although it is possible to catch up on some missed growth, long periods of poor nutrition and/or active inflammation may permanently stunt growth.

Of course, this can be a particularly difficult problem as food can exacerbate symptoms in people with active IBD and, similarly, decreasing food intake can sometimes improve symptoms. In Chapter 12, we discussed some strategies that may help. We also emphasized the importance of involving a qualified dietician. They can advise on dietary changes that may help to control symptoms, without compromising on calories and nutrients. Realistically, it is sometimes simply a case of encouraging children to eat as much as possible of whatever they feel like eating, regardless of its nutritional value! Sometimes, therefore, nutritional supplements are used to help boost the diet. These can even be given as a nasogastric feed at night. In very rare circumstances, intravenous feeding can be used (see Chapter 12).

Specific problems and questions

Immunizations

There is no reason why most children with IBD should not have the full schedule of immunizations, in fact, it is extremely important for them to do so. However, if a child is unwell at the time, they may miss scheduled immunizations, which should be given at a later date.

Another cause of missed immunizations in children with IBD relates to concern about the safety of vaccines in people taking immunosuppressive medication (including corticosteroids). With the exception of live vaccines (MMR, varicella zoster, oral polio, oral typhoid, yellow fever, and BCG) there is no need for concern about vaccinations in people taking immunosuppressants. Fortunately, most live vaccines are administered to people at an age at which IBD is unusual and use of immunosuppressants is extremely rare. As an alternative, some live vaccines (polio and typhoid) have alternative forms that are not live and are therefore safe.

Depression

Just like adults, children can become depressed. In children with IBD this is normally either a direct result of active disease, or of their medication. Steroids, for example, can have a marked psychological effect on people. Parents and healthcare professionals should be reassuring and supportive as, fortunately, depressive symptoms normally pass as the disease becomes less active or the medication is withdrawn. Discussing these symptoms with someone on the team is important. Occasionally psychologists or counsellors may be helpful and, rarely, antidepressant medication may be needed.

Is physical activity and sport safe?

Not only is it safe, but it is an important part of growing up and should not be avoided due to IBD. Having said this, there are several things to bear in mind. For example, there may well be times when a child is simply too fatigued or unwell to take part in physical activity. Allowing children with active IBD not to take part in physical activity when they feel unable to do so is as important as not preventing them from taking part when they wish to. Modifying physical activity, particularly during compulsory PE at school, may also be necessary at times. Most children know what they feel capable of doing, although it is important to remember that the desire to take part fully, particularly in team sports, can be very strong. This can occasionally lead to children pushing themselves too far.

Physical activity can make people need to open their bowels. This can be more pronounced in people with IBD. Finally, a proportion of people with IBD also have arthritis, which can limit their activity even when their IBD is well controlled.

Smoking

Adolescence is a time when young people experiment. Although it is very hard to stop young people experimenting with smoking, it is important that they understand the potential effects this may have on their IBD. For a young person with Crohn's disease, the knowledge that smoking increases the risk of needing an operation may be a greater deterrent than the often ignored general health risks.

Leaving home

Most people leave home in their late teens or early twenties. Many go on to college or university, or go travelling, while others may start families of their own.

Of course, having IBD does not prevent any of these things although, for some people, a little advance planning may be sensible. For example, if you are going travelling, or are planning to work abroad it is important to make sure that you have adequate supplies of medication. You may also need to make arrangements for monitoring of your treatment while you are away. Having someone to contact in case of a flare-up is also important. Fortunately, good IBD care is available almost worldwide. If your doctor is unable to recommend someone for you to see in your chosen destination, local patient groups are a good source of information. Of course, it is important to establish whether you will have to pay for care abroad and to consider carefully insurance options before you depart.

Similarly, if you are going to university or college, or are moving to a different area, it is wise to discuss this with your specialist first. This allows them to contact a local colleague in advance and to provide them with all the necessary information to allow your care to be transferred either temporarily or permanently.

Dealing with inflammatory bowel disease as a family

Having a child with IBD can be as much of a challenge for the parents and siblings as it can be for the person themselves (albeit in a different way!). Finding the balance between being supportive and overprotective can be extremely difficult. This is particularly true during adolescence. All children need to become independent as they grow older. Encouraging them, for example, to take control of their own medication and to learn about their condition may help them to go through the transition of child with IBD to adult with IBD.

Rebellion is a normal part of adolescence for many teenagers. Unfortunately, for people with IBD, this may take the form of rebellion against their disease. For example, some people go through a period of denial about their condition or stop taking medication. Alternatively, they may stop reporting symptoms to avoid being given medications, particularly if they dislike their side-effects. Remember that adolescence is a time when appearance and acceptance by our peers is of enormous importance. It is hardly surprising, therefore, that steroids, which can cause acne, weight gain, and a change in facial features, are often avoided by teenagers at all cost. Rarely, teenage girls with IBD deliberately use their condition to control their weight, rather like an eating disorder.

The relationship, therefore, between a young person with IBD and their medical team is of paramount importance—they must be able to trust and talk openly and honestly to the people who are looking after them.

Peer group support can be extremely helpful for teenagers with IBD. The opportunity to talk to someone else going through exactly the same things may be invaluable. Alternatively, slightly older people who have been through adolescence and have 'come out the other side' may also be a valuable source of support and knowledge.

Finally, it is important, although not necessarily easy, to prevent IBD becoming the central component of family life. Remember that brothers and sisters of a child with IBD may feel neglected and resentful if all the attention is focused on the affected child.

Support for young people with inflammatory bowel disease and their families

As well as the support group for children with IBD (CICRA), many patient organizations have sections specifically for younger people. For example, in the UK, the ia (Young ia), the NACC (Smilie's Network), and PINNT (the patient support group for people on nutritional support—Half PINNT) all have sections specifically for young people. In addition, local support groups can put you in touch with other people and families who are in a similar situation and who may be able to help or offer advice. Don't forget, however lonely you may feel, there is someone else out there who is going through the same things that you are. Talking with someone, who really understands through first-hand experience, can be very helpful. You might also be able to help them.

 Patient's perspective

Emma* was recently diagnosed with Crohn's disease aged 17. This is what she wrote:

> 'When I was first diagnosed with Crohn's I felt scared and as if I was the only person in the world to be in this position. No matter how much the doctors and nurses told me I would feel better I did not believe it. I was in a lot of pain and felt so tired. Worst of all, my hair was falling out. Once I started treatment, my life changed. From the first day I felt better. For the first time in a long time I had energy, an appetite and I felt my life was worth living again. Most important of all, I feel totally normal again.'

*Name changed.

Conclusions

IBD in children is effectively the same disease as it is in adults. It is investigated and treated in a very similar way in people of all ages. However, IBD presents different challenges when it affects young people; children are not simply small adults. In particular, attention needs to be paid to growth and development. It is important to consider the social and educational challenges faced by children and adolescents with IBD.

However, children are in general very resilient, often more so than adults, and can cope with enormous adversity. Also, while it is true that children can be very cruel to their peers they are also often very accepting and understanding. Finally, the role of the family is to support each other and to be understanding, without allowing IBD to take over family life.

16

Fertility and pregnancy in inflammatory bowel disease

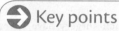

> ## Key points
>
> ◆ Inflammatory bowel disease affects many people during their reproductive years.
>
> ◆ The condition itself and its treatments, both medical and surgical, have the potential to affect the processes of reproduction.
>
> ◆ Controlling disease activity during pregnancy is important.
>
> ◆ Many drugs used to treat inflammatory bowel disease are considered safe in pregnancy.

Inflammatory bowel disease (IBD) commonly first presents in young people often before they have even thought about having a family. However, questions regarding fertility and pregnancy are among the most commonly asked by people with IBD. Because this is such an important and common issue, a lot of research has been done in the area. This means that many of the questions have clear answers.

Puberty

In children with IBD puberty can be delayed. During phases of active disease, growth is also delayed. When the disease is controlled and nutrition improves patients will usually grow and go through puberty normally (see Chapter 15). This does not lead to decreased fertility later in life.

Female fertility

Overall, women with IBD have similar rates of infertility as the general population (about 1 in 10). Female fertility is not impaired by ulcerative colitis except in women who have had surgery (see below) or during active disease. In women with significant flare-ups of disease activity, ovulation and menstruation can become irregular.

By contrast, research has shown that women with Crohn's disease have fewer children after diagnosis than would be expected, suggesting that they have decreased fertility. This is probably only the case for severe Crohn's disease and many studies show normal fertility in women with mild or controlled Crohn's disease.

Pouch surgery and conception

Studies have shown that women who have had pouch surgery have fewer successful pregnancies than women who have not had surgery. This is probably due to the effects of complex surgery in the pelvis causing scarring. This can affect the normal processes required for conception, for example, by blocking the fallopian tubes. Egg production by the ovaries remains healthy. Instead, the problem seems to be with the passage of the egg into the uterus for fertilization. Fortunately, therefore, in most cases successful pregnancy can be achieved by in vitro fertilization (IVF).

Effects of drug treatment on female fertility

None of the drugs used in IBD appears to have an adverse effect on a woman's ability to conceive. In fact, because having active disease reduces fertility, drugs that control disease activity may increase the chance of becoming pregnant. However, that is not to say that all drugs are safe to use in pregnancy (see below).

Contraception

The oral contraceptive pill may not be fully absorbed in people who have bad diarrhoea and, therefore, women with IBD should not rely exclusively on it for safe contraception especially when they are having a flare-up.

Male fertility

Sulfasalazine can cause reduced numbers of healthy sperm. This improves a few weeks after the drug is stopped. Other aminosalicylates, for example mesalazine, do not affect male fertility. Active disease does not appear to decrease fertility in men.

Living with the disease: sex and inflammatory bowel disease

There are a few reasons why having IBD can interfere with a normal sex life. These include IBD or medication causing a lack of libido. More specifically, the IBD itself may interfere directly with people's enjoyment of sex.

Some people have particular concerns about body image. Embarrassment about scars, perianal disease, or a stoma can make it hard to relax and may make people worried about being naked with their partner. Of course, it is easier if you feel you know your partner well enough to discuss your concerns. They will almost certainly understand.

Some women with IBD may get pain deep inside during intercourse due to inflammation of small bowel loops in the pelvis. This is called dyspareunia. Treating active disease will usually improve this symptom. Similarly, previous surgery can alter the position of the organs in the pelvis, which may make sex uncomfortable. Trying different positions may help. Rarely, surgical procedures may cause damage to nerves in the pelvis. For women this may alter clitoral sensation while for men it may result in erectile or ejaculatory problems. Fortunately there is a variety of treatments available for erectile dysfunction.

Perianal abscesses or fistulae can make intercourse uncomfortable. Lubricating jelly can help as will treatment of the underlying disease. Receptive anal intercourse may be best avoided if you have active perianal abscesses or fistulation.

It is always worth asking for advice from your specialist or IBD nurse (however embarrassing that may seem) as they may be able to reassure you and help you overcome some of your fears. Finally it is worth remembering that there are many other ways of being intimate with a loved one than having sex.

Outcome of pregnancy

The majority of research shows that the outcome of pregnancy in women with inactive IBD is the same as for the general population. In other words, if the IBD is well controlled during pregnancy, there is no increased risk of miscarriage, premature delivery, or congenital abnormalities.

However, there appears to be an increased rate of miscarriage and premature delivery when IBD is not well controlled during pregnancy. Underweight newborn babies are also more common if the mother's IBD was poorly controlled during pregnancy. It is important, therefore, to ensure, as much as possible, that IBD is in remission before considering pregnancy.

Planning to get pregnant? Think ahead . . .

First of all you should try to get your IBD well controlled. This might require drugs or sometimes even surgery. You should also make sure you are eating properly and taking folic acid supplements. If you smoke, you should stop, and, if you drink, you should decrease your alcohol intake.

Many people with IBD need drugs to maintain their disease in remission. Considering trying for a baby is *NOT* the time to stop taking medication. This increases your chances of a flare-up and might have damaging effects on the pregnancy. We would recommend discussing things with your team (consultant, GP, or IBD nurse) well in advance, even if pregnancy is not something you are planning immediately. It's worth knowing what you plan to do with respect to drug treatment if you become pregnant. It also helps if you have a comfortable knowledge of the risks and benefits of continuing your medication versus getting a flare-up.

In an ideal world all pregnancies would be planned, though as we all know, life does not always go according to plan. However, it is worth taking precautions against pregnancy during flare-ups of disease and waiting until the disease is better before stopping contraception.

Finally, don't panic if you become pregnant unexpectedly or have a flare-up of your disease during pregnancy. Simply contact your gastroenterologist and obstetrician; the chances of this resulting in a major problem with your baby are still very small.

Safety of drugs during pregnancy

One of the biggest dilemmas faced by women with IBD who are planning a family is whether to continue with maintenance drug treatment during pregnancy and breast feeding. Because IBD is common in women of childbearing age, we now have a lot of information to help people make their decisions. The risks of continuing medication must be weighed against the risks of getting a flare-up if you stop them.

Aminosalicylates

These can be used safely during pregnancy and breast-feeding. There is no danger to the baby if you are taking these drugs. However, although all women should take folic acid before conception and during early pregnancy, this is particularly important for women taking sulfasalazine.

Steroids

There is probably a weak association between the use of steroids in pregnancy and a (very) slightly increased risk of cleft palate. However, it is clear that the risks to the unborn child are much greater if active disease is left untreated. Therefore, if your disease flares up during pregnancy, it is much safer for your baby if you take a course of steroids than if you continue through pregnancy with active disease.

Immunosuppressants

Azathioprine and 6 mercaptopurine can also be used during pregnancy. Although theoretically they may alter the development of an embryo, this does not seem to happen in the large majority of studies that have looked at pregnancy outcome in women taking azathioprine or mercaptopurine. If there is an increased risk to unborn babies it is very small

Therefore, if your disease is well controlled by azathioprine but was difficult to control before you started it, your doctor may recommend you consider continuing it during pregnancy. Again, this is because it is safer for your baby if your disease remains controlled.

Methotrexate causes fetal abnormalities and should be avoided by both men and women contemplating becoming parents for at least 6 months before conception. It should be avoided by women throughout pregnancy and breast-feeding.

Biologics

Infliximab is not recommended during pregnancy because of lack of knowledge about its effect. However recent results from Belgium where they followed 22 pregnancies in which the mother had infliximab, have shown that there were no bad effects on mother, delivery, or baby. In this group infliximab was avoided during the last trimester (3 months before delivery) when it crosses the placenta. Because infliximab and other similar drugs are being used more and more to keep symptoms of Crohn's disease under control there will be increasing experience of their use in pregnancy. At the moment we would recommend that you take advice from an expert in managing IBD. Your own doctor will be happy to refer you to an expert if your condition is complicated and you want to get pregnant.

There is very little information on which to base an opinion on the use of **adalimumab** during pregnancy. It is classified as low risk according to results from animal studies but human data are very limited. It is likely (but not definite) that the risks of using adalimumab will be similar to those for infliximab.

Antibiotics

Metronidazole is probably safe. It has not been associated with an increased risk of birth defects, preterm delivery or miscarriage. The majority of data about its use in pregnancy comes from people who received short courses (5–7 days). There is limited information about longer exposure during pregnancy.

Ciprofloxacin has not been associated with problems in humans but animal studies show an increased risk of joint problems in the fetus. Again human data comes from people who have taken short courses and cannot necessarily be extrapolated to longer treatment as is often used in IBD or pouchitis.

Antidiarrhoeals

Loperamide appears safe in both animals and humans. There is less information available for lomotil. It is not known whether lomotil crosses the placenta and human studies have not been done. Therefore, its use is not recommended in pregnancy.

Safety of drugs in men fathering children

As mentioned above, sulfasalazine may reduce fertility in men. However, if the partner of a man taking sulfasalazine becomes pregnant, there do not appear to be any adverse outcomes. Other 5-aminosalicylic acids are also safe. The vast majority of data suggest that azathioprine and mercaptopurine are safe. Methotrexate should be avoided for 6 months prior to conception. It is clearly teratogenic if taken by women and, although there is not much information for men who father children while taking methotrexate, the theoretical risks are very off-putting and it should therefore be avoided. Data on other drugs are very limited.

Effect of pregnancy on your inflammatory bowel disease

If your disease is in remission it will be likely to stay that way during pregnancy. If your disease is active, pregnancy is unlikely to change the activity.

Can I have a normal delivery?

Most patients with IBD will be able to have a normal delivery. In some patients who have had previous pouch surgery or surgery for perianal disease, it is possible your surgeon would recommend that you do not have a normal vaginal delivery. This will be to protect you from the possible effects of trauma to the anal canal during delivery. This can lead to future problems with continence.

Antenatal care

It is sensible to book an appointment with your gastroenterologist before trying to become pregnant. When you do become pregnant you should let

Keep in touch . . .

When you are pregnant it is very important to keep in close contact with your IBD healthcare team. It is important that you are seen and treated early if you suffer a flare-up. If you do have a flare-up contact your IBD team as soon as possible. Your treatment options will be discussed carefully and sensitively with you. You are more likely to have problems with your pregnancy if you decide not to see a doctor because of concerns about being given drugs. Options such as topical therapy, elemental diet, and other totally safe treatments might be appropriate. No one will make you do anything you don't want to, but it is important that you make your decisions based on sensible evidence-based advice from experts.

Table 16.1

Drugs and breast feeding	Recommendation	Side-effect
Mesalazine	OK	Rarely diarrhoea in infant
Sulfasalazine	OK	Rarely diarrhoea in infant
Corticosteroids	OK	
Azathioprine/mercaptopurine	Not recommended	Not known
Methotrexate	Not recommended	Risk of cancer
Infliximab	Probably OK—limited data	
Ciprofloxacin	Not recommended	Not known
Metronidazole	Not recommended	Not known
Loperamide	Not recommended	May affect lactation

your medical team know. When you book for antenatal care you need to make sure that you tell the midwife or obstetrician about your IBD. You should also give them details of your gastroenterologist. The teams will then work together with you to ensure that you have a healthy pregnancy and healthy baby.

Conclusions

IBD should not affect your ability to have a family; however, active disease can decrease a woman's chance of becoming pregnant. Active disease during pregnancy is also known to increase the risks to the unborn child; therefore, it is safer for some patients to continue their normal medication while pregnant to control their disease. Fortunately most drugs used to control IBD appear to be safe in pregnancy. Most importantly, you should discuss any concerns you have with your specialist before trying for a baby.

Appendix 1

Patient support groups

United Kingdom

NACC—National Association of Colitis and Crohn's Disease

4 Beaumont House, Sutton Road, St Albans, Herts, AL1 5HH
Tel: +44 1727 844296
Information line: 0845 130 2233/
http://www.nacc.org.uk

CICRA—Crohn's in Childhood Research Association

Parkgate House, 356 West Barnes Lane, Motspur Park, Surrey, VT3 6NB
Tel: 020 8949 6209
http://www.cicra.org

ia—the ileostomy and internal pouch support group

Peverill House, 1–5 Mill Road, Ballyclare, Co. Antrim, BT39 9DR
Tel: 0800 0184 724 (free) or +44 28 9334 4043
http://www.iasupport.org

Young ia

c/o IA National Office Peverill House, 1–5 Mill Road, Ballyclare, BT39 9DR
Tel: 0800 0184724
http://www.youngia.org.uk

PINNT—Patients on Intravenous and Nasogastric Nutrition Therapy

Half PINNT (young members)
PO Box 3126, Christchurch Dorset, BH23 2XS
http://www.pinnt.com

PSC Support

39 Belvoir Road, London, SE22 0QY
Tel: +44 20 8693 8789
http://www.psc-support.demon.co.uk

International inflammatory bowel disease patient support groups

Algeria

Association des Porteurs de Maladies Inflammatoires Chroniques d'Intestin
de la Wilaya d'Oran
http://www.afa.asso.fr/algerie

Australia

Australian Crohn's and Colitis Association (ACCA)
http://www.acca.net.au

Austria

Österreichische Morbus Crohn/Colitis Ulcerosa Vereinigung (ÖMCCV)
http://www.oemccv.at

Belgium

Crohn en Colitis Ulcerosa Vereniging vzw (CCV)
http://www.ccv-vzw.be

Brazil

Association Brazilia Colitis Ulcerosa & Crohns (ABCD)
http://www.abcd.org.br

Canada

Crohn's and Colitis Foundation of Canada (CCFC)
http://www.ccfc.ca

Croatia

Hrvatsko Udruzenje za Crohnovu Bolest i Ulcerozni Kolitis (HUCUK)
http://www.hucuk.hr

Cyprus

Pancyprian Associatin of Ulcerative Colitis and Crohn's (CYCCA)
PO Box 27553 Nicosia, Cyprus, 2430

Czech Republic

Crocodile (CROhn and COlitis DILEtants)
Crocodile CZ, Jirovcova 24, 37004 Ceske Budejovice, Czech Republic

Denmark

Colitis-Crohn Foreningen (CCF)
http://www.ccf.dk

Europe

EFCCA—European Federation of Crohn's and Ulcerative Colitis Association
http://www.efcca.org

Finland

Crohn jz Colitis ry (CCAFIN)
http://www.crohnjacolitis.fi

Germany

Deutsche Morbus Crohn/Colitis Ulcerova Vereinigung (DCCV e.V.)
http://www.dccv.de

Hungary

Magyarorszagi Crohn-Colitises Betegek Egyesulete (MCCBE)
http://www.mccbe.hu

Iceland

Crohn's og Colitis Ulcerosa Samtökin (CCU-Samtökin)
http://www.ccu.is

Ireland

Irish Society for Colitis and Crohn's Disease (ISCC)
http://www.iscc.ie

Israel

The Israel Foundation for Crohn's Disease and Ulcerative Colitis
PO Box 5231, Herzlia, Israel

Italy

Aoociazione per la Malattie Infiammatorie Croniche dell'Intestino (AMICI)
http://www.amiciitalia.org

Japan

IBD Patients Network
http://www.ibdnetwork.org

Luxembourg

Association Luxembourgeoise de la Maladie de Crohn (ALMC)
http://www.afa.assoc.fr/luxembourg

Morocco

Association Marocaine pour le Soutien des Malades Atteints de la Recto-
Colite Ulcéro-Hémorragique et de la Maladie de Crohn
http://www.afa.asso.fr/maroc

The Netherlands

Crohn en Colitis Ulcerosa Vereniging Nederland (CCUVN)
http://www.crohn-colitis.nl

New Zealand

Crohns and Colitis Support Group—CCSG
http://www.ccsg.org.nz

Norway

Landsforeningen mot Fordøyelsessykdommer (LMF)
http://www.lmfnorge.no

Portugal

Associacao Portuguesa da Doenca Inflamatoria do Intestino (APDI)
http://www.apdi.org.pt

Slovakia

Slovak Crohn Club (VUV (SCC))
http://www.crohnclub.sk

Slovenia

Društvo za KVCB (SAIBD)
http://www.kvcb.si

South Africa

South African Crohn's and Colitis Association (SACCA)
http://www.ccsg.org.za

Spain

Asociacion de Enformos de Crohn y Colitis Ulcerosa (ACCU)
http://www.accuesp.com

Sweden

Riksförbundet för Magoch Tarmsjuka (RMT)
http://www.magotarm.se

Switzerland

Schweizerische Morbus Crohn/Colitis Ulcerosa Vereinigung (SMCCV)
http://www.smccv.ch (German); http://www.asmcc.ch (French)

USA

Crohn's and Colitis Foundation of America (CCFA)
http://www.ccfa.org

Zimbabwe

Zimbabwe Association for Colitis & Crohn's Disease, 2 Montclaire Close,
Borrowdale, Harare, Zimbabwe

Glossary

A

5-ASA: 5-aminosalicylic acid. A drug used to treat IBD

Abscess: an abnormal cavity containing pus

Acute: short lasting

Anaemia: deficiency of haemoglobin leading to inefficient carriage of oxygen in the blood

Anastomosis: surgical join between two pieces of bowel

Ankylosing spondylitis: a type of arthritis affecting the joints between the bones of the spine

Antibody: a molecule produced by the immune system when it encounters something foreign

Appendix: a small pocket of bowel attached to the caecum

Arthritis: inflammation of joints causing pain and swelling

Axial arthritis: arthritis affecting the axial skeleton, that is the spine and pelvis

Azathioprine: an immunosuppressive drug used to treat IBD

B

B12: a vitamin absorbed in the last part of the small bowel

Balsalazide: a 5-ASA drug

Biologics: a new group of drugs used in IBD that specifically target part of the inflammatory response. Examples include infliximab and adalimumab

C

CAM: Complementary and alternative medicine. Medical practices not covered by conventional medicine

Capsule endoscope: a small pill containing a camera that is swallowed and takes pictures as it passes through the small bowel

Carbohydrate: an energy source in food. Includes sugars and starches. Carbohydrates are produced by plants

Chronic: long lasting

Cirrhosis: irreversible scarring of the liver caused by chronic liver disease

Colectomy: operation to remove some or all of the colon

Colon: large bowel, large intestine

Colonoscopy: an endoscopic examination of the large bowel and terminal ileum

Colovesical fistula: fistula from large bowel to bladder

CRP (C-reactive protein): a protein in the blood often found at higher concentrations during flares of IBD

CT (computed tomography) scan: an X-ray scan of the internal organs of the body

Cyclosporine: an immunosuppressant drug used in acute severe colitis

Cytokines: small chemical compounds that circulate in the blood stream when there is inflammation or infection in the body

D

Defecation: passing faeces, opening bowels, passing stool, number twos, pooing

DEXA scan: a scan that measures the density of bones. The results are compared with values for the general population to estimate risk of fractures

Digestion: the processing of food by our guts into absorbable nutrients

Distal colitis: (left-sided colitis) inflammation of the rectum, sigmoid and descending colon

Dysentery: an infection causing diarrhoea (often bloody) and fever

Dyspareunia: pain in the pelvis felt during sexual intercourse

E

Elemental feed: a feed consisting of all the basic components of diet in simple forms

Endoscopy: an examination to view part of the gut using a flexible tube containing a camera. Sometimes endoscopy is used to mean gastroscopy

Enema: a foam or liquid containing a drug that is delivered to the bowel through the anus

Enteral feeding: supplemental feeding into the gut, normally through a tube

Enterocutaneous fistula: fistula from bowel to abdominal wall

Enteroenteric fistula: fistula from bowel to bowel

Enteroscopy: an endoscopic examination of the small bowel

ESR (erythrocyte sedimentation rate): a blood test used to see if IBD is active

Extensive colitis: pancolitis, total colitis; inflammation of the entire colon and rectum

F

Faeces: stools, bowel motions, poo, number twos

FBC (full blood count, aka CBC—complete blood count). A blood test that measures the haemoglobin, white cell count, and platelet count

Ferritin: a protein in the blood that is measured to detect iron deficiency

Fibre: indigestible carbohydrate that adds bulk to stool and helps to keep it soft

Fissure: a small tear in the skin lining the anal canal which can cause bleeding. Can be very painful when passing motions

Fistula: an abnormal channel causing a connection between two surfaces that are not normally linked (e.g. gut lumen and skin)

Flare up: a worsening of symptoms of colitis or Crohn's disease especially when going from remission into active disease

Flatus: wind, farts

Flexible sigmoidoscopy: an endoscopic examination of the rectum, sigmoid colon, and descending colon

Folate: a vitamin absorbed in the first part of the small bowel found in leafy vegetables

Frequency: the need to open your bowels more often than usual

Fructose: a sugar in the diet. May cause diarrhoea, abdominal pain, and bloating in some people

Functional symptoms: symptoms not caused by inflammation

G

Gastroscopy. (OGD) Endoscopy of the oesophagus, stomach, and duodenum

Gene: a piece of DNA that defines one of our characteristic. Everyone has about 30 000 different genes

Growth chart: a chart used to plot the height and weight of children to ensure they are growing

Gut: alimentary tract, digestive tract, bowel, gastrointestinal tract

H

HPN (home parenteral nutrition): using intravenous nutrition (TPN) at home

I

IBS: irritable bowel syndrome. A functional gut disorder that causes a change in bowel habit and abdominal pain

Ileocaecal valve: the join between the end of the ileum and the caecum

Ileostomy: surgically created opening of the ileum onto the abdominal wall. The bowel contents are delivered into a bag (hence ileostomy bag)

Infertility: reduced ability to achieve natural conception of an embryo

Inflammation: swelling, redness, pain, and heat. Inflammation leads to tissue destruction and is followed by attempts at repair

Immunization: the use of vaccines to make people immune to a variety of infections

Intravenous: into a vein. An injection. An infusion of a drug or nutrition

Intramuscular injection: injection into a muscle

J

Jaundice: a yellow discoloration of the skin caused by increased concentration of a bile pigment in the blood

L

Lactose: a sugar in the diet. May cause diarrhoea, abdominal pain, and bloating in some people

LFTs: liver function (blood) tests

Lumen: the inside of the gut tube

M

Maintenance therapy: drug treatment used to keep IBD in remission

Malabsorption: failure of the effective transfer of nutrients from the lumen across the gut wall into the body

MAP (*Mycobacterium avium* subspecies *paratuberculosis*): an organism that causes a disease similar to Crohn's disease in cattle

MDT (multidisciplinary team): the team of healthcare professionals who, in combination, provide care for people with IBD

(6-)Mercaptopurine: an immunosuppressant drug very similar to azathioprine used as maintenance therapy in IBD

Mesalazine (mesalamine): 5-ASA

Methotrexate: an immunosuppressant drug used as a maintenance therapy in Crohn's disease and sometimes in ulcerative colitis

MMR: a vaccine given to children to prevent measles, mumps, and rubella. Has not been shown to cause Crohn's disease

MRI (magnetic resonance imaging): a scan of the internal organs of the body using strong magnets rather than X-rays

Mucosa: the thin inner layer of the wall of the gut. The mucosa lines the lumen of the gut

Mucus: a jelly-like substance produced by the bowel

N

Nasogastric tube: a very small tube inserted through the nose into the stomach. It is used either to drain the stomach contents in patients with obstruction, or to allow enteral feeding

NSAIDs (non-steroidal anti-inflammatory drugs): e.g. ibuprofen, diclofenac. Anti-inflammatory painkillers, often used for arthritis. Can cause flares of IBD in some people

Nutritional therapy: a form of treatment for Crohn's disease in which the only nutrition taken is in the form of elemental or polymeric liquid feed

O

Obstruction: blockage of bowel often caused by stricturing

Oesophagus: food pipe, gullet

OGD – see gastroscopy

Olsalazine: a 5-ASA drug

Oral: By mouth. A route for taking medication. Or, of the mouth. E.g. oral Crohn's disease

Osteoporosis: thinning of the bones causing them to become weak and more prone to fracture

Ovum: egg produced by the ovaries

P

Paediatrician: a doctor who specializes in looking after children

Parasite: an organism that lives in or on another organism, the host. The parasite gets its nutrition from the host

Parenteral feeding: feed given directly into the bloodstream. Intravenous nutrition

Perforation: a hole or leak in gut wall

perianal abscess/fistula: an abscess/fistula that opens around the anus

Peritonitis: inflammation of the lining of the internal cavity of the abdomen usually caused by a perforation of the bowel

Placebo: a dummy drug used in drug trials

Polymeric feed: similar to an elemental feed

Pouch: a surgically constructed reservoir made from small intestine attached to the anus after colectomy

Prebiotic: a substance that is taken by mouth that encourages the growth of bacteria in the bowel that may improve health

Probiotic: bacteria taken by mouth that may improve health

Proctitis: inflammation of the rectum

Proctocolectomy: operation to remove the entire colon and rectum

Protein: molecules in food that provide amino acids. An essential part of the diet

Puberty: the physical changes that occur in body shape, body hair, and sexual organs when children become adults

R

Rectal examination: an internal examination of the anal canal and rectum using a gloved finger with lubricant jelly

Rectovaginal fistula: a fistula from rectum to vagina

Relapse: active disease

Remission: inactive disease

Right hemicolectomy: operation to remove the terminal ileum and caecum

Rigid sigmoidoscopy: an examination of the rectum using an inflexible plastic or metal tube inserted through the anus

S

Sacroiliac joints: the joints between the pelvis and the spine

Seton: loop of thread or rubber tubing passed along a fistula to allow drainage of pus and prevent abscess formation

Short bowel syndrome (intestinal failure): A condition in which much of the small bowel has been removed so that it is not possible to absorb adequate nutrients from food

Small bowel: intestine, small intestine. Consists of duodenum jejunum and ileum

Steroids: aka corticosteroids. Powerful anti-inflammatory drugs used to induce remission in IBD

Stool chart: a chart recording frequency and consistency of bowel motions

Stricture: a narrowing of the bowel lumen due to bowel wall thickening or scarring

Stricturoplasty: operation to open up a narrowing in the bowel without resecting any of it

Subcutaneous injection: an injection under the skin

Subtotal colitis: inflammation of the rectum, sigmoid, descending and transverse colon

Suppository: a drug that is placed into the rectum through the anus

T

Teratogenic: capable of causing birth defects

Thiopurine: collective term for 6-mercaptopurine and azathioprine

TPMT (thiopurine methyltransferase): an enzyme involved in the metabolism of thiopurines. The activity of this enzyme varies from person to person and can be measured by a blood test. The test is often done, before starting one of these drugs

Topical treatment: drug treatment that works by being in direct contact with the area of inflammation. In IBD this usually refers to suppositories and enemas

TPN (total parenteral nutrition): giving all nutrition intravenously

Trichuris suis: a parasitic worm that normally infects pigs. Currently being investigated as a treatment for IBD

U

U+Es (urea and electrolytes): a blood test chiefly testing kidney function

Ulcer: a break in the lining of the gut, mouth, or skin

Urgency: the need to get to the toilet quickly

W

White blood cells: the cells in the blood that fight infection. They are also responsible for causing inflammation

Index